THRIVE

A PRACTICAL GUIDE TO HARNESS YOUR RESILIENCE AND REALISE YOUR POTENTIAL

RICHARD SUTTON

THRIVE

A PRACTICAL GUIDE TO HARNESS YOUR RESILIENCE AND REALISE YOUR POTENTIAL

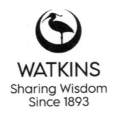

WATKINS
Sharing Wisdom
Since 1893

Content warning: this book contains some descriptions of physical and emotional abuse

First published in 2023
by Pan Macmillan South Africa
This edition published in 2024 by
Watkins, an imprint of Watkins Media Limited
Unit 11, Shepperton House
89-93 Shepperton Road
London
N1 3DF

enquiries@watkinspublishing.com

Design and typography copyright © Watkins Media Limited 2024

Text Copyright © Richard Sutton 2024

1 3 5 7 9 10 8 6 4 2

Designed and typeset by JCS Publishing Services Ltd.

Printed and bound in the UK by TJ Books Ltd.

A CIP record for this book is available from the British Library

ISBN: 978-1-78678-850-4 (Hardback)
ISBN: 978-1-78678-868-9 (eBook)

www.watkinspublishing.com

Dedicated to those who have had to face and overcome struggles and adversity, and who are supporting others in their journey.

CONTENTS

Part 3: Lessons in resilience from Olympic champions – a masterclass in behavioural science

INTRODUCTION

Imbedded in the challenge is the gift.

Thirty-five years ago I would not have agreed with this statement, but looking back I realise and appreciate how true this statement really is.

It was a fairly normal summer's morning in Johannesburg. The sky was clear, things were peaceful and it was warm outside. My younger brother and I were up a little before 7am (we shared a room) and soon started talking, playing and laughing. Without warning, the door burst open and my stepfather stormed in. He was a short man, with a violent temper and very fragile ego. Unfortunately, our play and laughter had woken him up. He wasn't there to ask us to be quiet but to ensure that it never happened again. He began to discipline me with his favourite bamboo cane, striking me repeatedly like a practiced samurai for my perceived offence – disturbing his sleep. Fortunately for him, the welts were predominantly on my back so they would be fairly easy to hide.

I was in a lot of pain and struggling to get dressed, move freely and sit down. Knowing that it would draw attention from teachers, I was instructed to say that I had fallen. I fearfully followed the instructions but the teachers didn't buy into it and asked me to lift my shirt. Their shared eye contact said everything there was to say. I'm positive that if this were to happen today I would be removed from my home environment, but back then, in the late 1970s, things were kept quiet.

What made this particular event unusual was not the physical or psychological trauma, as this was unfortunately a fairly common occurrence, but rather that the incident took place in the morning.

Like many children, I grew up in a home that was afflicted by alcohol abuse. Living in this environment meant that the evenings were more likely to be the time when abuse was commonly meted out. I used to dread 5pm as this was when the wine or spirits would come out and the cycle of hostility and conflict would begin. At first the drinking was fairly moderate, perhaps even a little festive, but with increasing consumption the verbal battles began and more often than not some form of trauma would invariably unfold. Visits to the hospital emergency room were not uncommon for joint dislocations, lacerations or even severe bruising.

As a young child, I was often caught in the middle of the crossfire between my parents and was a soft target for the offloading of anger, resentment and aggression.

When I got home from school every day and walked in the house my heart would start to pound, my palms began to sweat and my breathing became shallow. I had to be on high alert as I didn't know what was waiting for me; seldom was it good.

This struggle was further compounded by the stress of significant financial challenges in the home. We seldom stayed in a house for more than a year or two, either due to bank repossession or eviction for not paying the rent. This meant that any form of additional expense such as an extra after-school activity, sports equipment or even stationery for school was not affordable. At the same time, I would change schools a total of seven times over my school career and had to endure the accompanying stresses and challenges, not to mention the lack of friends and long-term relationships.

I did my best to stay away from the house during the day by hanging out in the park and riding my bike for hours, but my main aim was to stay away for as long as I could at night.

By the age of 13, I had found a job as a waiter. While it wasn't legal to work at that age, I looked older due to the chronic stress I dealt with. Finally, I had found a routine that kept me safe. I would leave for school at 7am every morning, amuse myself for a few hours in the afternoon, briefly return home and change for my shift at the restaurant and then head off to work and return at approximately 10.30pm, by which time things would be quiet and calm at home. I worked six days a week and continued to do so for the next five years. While this gave me financial freedom and removed me from the challenges in the home, it did mean that I sacrificed sleep, my personal health and any opportunities to pursue sports, and it cost me an education.

I barely managed to stay afloat at school. All I aimed for was the lowest mark possible that would prevent me from failing. That's what adversity does – it strips us of our dreams and any ambition.

Sitting in class every day, I felt completely lost. I was exhausted and replaying the traumatic events of my life over and over again. My classroom experience was dominated by constant dreams of a different reality.

Ironically, despite my struggle with all other subjects, I was particularly good at history as it required the repetition of facts and events. But any discipline that required systematic process or demanded homework would be particularly challenging for me. Today, I would probably be prescribed methylphenidate (Ritalin or Concerta) for attention-deficit disorder.

In a token attempt to salvage my academic woes, one of the schools suggested I complete an aptitude test to determine my areas of strength and weakness. I've realised that I loved receiving any kind of attention as interest in my wellbeing was fairly limited at home.

Through a collaborative effort, I was taken to see one of the best practitioners and I was so excited I could hardly contain myself. As a lost teenager I needed to hear what I would be good at as all I heard was what my inadequacies were. I walked into the practitioner's office, had a short discussion with him, filled out the necessary forms, performed some tests and tried to solve a few puzzles. Finally the time had come.

I would have a target to aim for, a purpose and a mission outside of basic survival. Unfortunately the assessment outcome was not good. The "expert" strongly believed that there was nothing I showed any aptitude for or towards and simply shook his head. I was gutted, but I had experienced so many failures and disappointments that I knew that was not going to be the last.

I, like so many children in the world, had become a victim of circumstance, powerless to change my reality.

During this time, I became intent on self-protection. There were times when I was able to take karate lessons for a month or two, but logistics (specifically needing a lift) and a lack of time would prevent me from taking it further. With the little formal training I had, I would practise for hours – punching, kicking, doing the basic katas and stretching. It was a tremendous comfort and a great source of confidence for me. Watching sport and the occasional martial arts movie would provide ongoing motivation in my world that appeared to be devoid of growth opportunities.

I felt a strong urgency to become physically stronger as strength was a powerful deterrent in the home I was growing up in. I began doing push-ups and sit-ups and I would exercise for hours on end in the gaps between school and work. Without any form of structure, guidance or equipment, I was my own teacher, motivator and mentor.

Needless to say, consistency, variety and progression were lacking, but I did the best I could under the trying circumstances. The larger struggle in my life at the time was not the abuse but the neglect as my life lacked any kind of support. This void was on an emotional level as well as in the form of practical assistance.

But everyone was trying their best under the circumstances and there were family members and even strangers who showed me kindness and care even when I was undeserving (I could be a handful at times), but it hardly compensated for the emptiness I was feeling inside.

To compound matters, decades later I discovered that I have several gene variants that increase my vulnerability to adversity by amplifying my reactivity to stress and limiting my ability to recover from traumatic events.

By the age of 18 I had learnt the value of hard work and commitment but lacked many other life skills. The tools and traits that had served me well included an outgoing personality (I was forced to be), being open to new experiences and agreeableness. What I sorely lacked was an environment that was positive, encouraging, caring, attentive and empathic. Moreover, I would see my many failures and setbacks as a personal reflection of me, from the vantage point of a victim, and I was always looking to be saved in some sense. My emotions governed my reality and this is something that has taken me years to repair. I had no way of controlling my stress responses or regulating myself following challenging events. Lastly, I had neglected my health. I had no informed sense of diet, nutritional supplements, regular exercise or other basic health behaviours.

I had resigned myself to a life of mediocrity. With a poor education, low resilience, no major skills or aptitudes and a limited support base, the world felt like a hard and lonely place. I tried to spend some time overseas before my compulsory national service in an attempt to start my life over, but my internal struggles followed me – I found no ease, fulfilment or joy.

However, the turning point was around the corner. The thing I feared the most – compulsory national service – turned out to be the catalyst for positive change. The initial experience was not a success and in fact was a disaster due to my limited fitness and poor mental strength, but there was a turning point after about two months and the experience became a perfect masterclass in resilience. I was taught my first major life skills, which included the power of grit, persistence and perseverance. That period of my life showed me the immense value of support and the strength of a team, as up until then I had always been alone. I learnt that we all need to be positively challenged to move forward in life. By far the two greatest lessons learnt were understanding the power of health behaviours and physical fitness in supporting our mental and emotional wellbeing, and the value of hope – the sincere belief that your life is going to be better in the future.

Finally, at the age of 20, I truly believed I could do anything I set my mind to.

While these are incredible resilience skills and were the genesis of a new chapter in my life, the struggles of the past still held me captive, especially on an emotional front. Poor formative education haunted me and I therefore found myself unable to study what I wanted, only what I could afford and what my academic achievements (or lack thereof) would allow.

Throughout my formative years what helped me to emotionally escape from the pain and sadness was the world of sport. Watching elite athletes perform the impossible and achieve excellence under the most demanding of circumstances gave me more than respite, it gave me a compass. As far fetched as it was at the time, somehow and in some context I wanted to share that reality. But circumstances, compounded by time, had eventually corroded all forms of confidence, hope and aspiration.

Yet I found myself entering my second decade of life better equipped and ready to reignite a dream, namely a life in professional sport. My intended role would be to support others in their athletic develoment and career path.

With the new skills I had acquired in the military I channelled all my resources into learning and educating myself; after all I had become my own greatest teacher. Learning from all sources and perspectives without limitation or restriction, my days, nights and weekends were dedicated to my former weakness but newfound strength – knowledge acquisition. My goal was to help the world's best athletes overcome their personal challenges and roadblocks.

I had a PhD in pain, failure, setbacks, disappointments and hurdles, which had all given me some incredible gifts. Empathy, compassion, heightened sensitivity and enhanced perceptual processes. This included the ability to predict the way people are going to move and their future actions. I was able to determine an opponent's levels of focus, confidence, competitiveness and intended actions.

Over the next two decades I continued adding to my repertoire of resilience skills, which included adaptability, consciousnesses and cognitive reappraisal – the most important trait of all.

What I came to realise is that we all have the ability to survive adversity and hardship. In fact, humans are hardwired for it. What defines resilience is not surviving but rather overcoming adversity. This reality is a learnt skill – a collection of behaviours and psychological traits that when unified allow us to realise our dreams and our fullest potential.

The intention of this book is to share those fundamental skills and provide you with the tools that will help you to better navigate the complexity that is life.

PART I

UNDERSTANDING OUR POTENTIAL

THE ULTIMATE STORY
OF RESILIENCE

Despite how we sometimes feel or what society and social norms instil in us, we are not defined by where our life journey begins, let alone the failures, disappointments or setbacks that happen along the way. Yet we tend to measure ourselves, our family, close friends and even businesses on established norms, big data, analytics, trend-lines and averages, with little wiggle room for error. So much so that if you're not hitting established milestones, conforming to the appropriate curve, beating unrealistic targets or living up to pre-existing expectations, it evokes in us worry, anxiety, fear and a profound sense of personal failure.

According to the Centers for Disease Control and Prevention,[1] by the age of three a child should be following instructions that include up to three steps. Additionally, they should be able to name most familiar things, carry a conversation using two to three sentences and robotically state age, name and gender. What does it mean for a child who falls below this established set of criteria? What are the implications for their parents? Are they destined for a life of mediocre accomplishments, hardships and overwhelming failings? As a parent, this is a thought process that can consume you and this I know from personal experience.

"The years of anxious searching in the dark, with their intense longing, their alternation of confidence and exhaustion and the final emergence into light — only those who have experienced it can understand it."

ALBERT EINSTEIN

THE REST IS HISTORY

The real-life story of Albert Einstein is one that perfectly illustrates the concept of resilience and how the failures, trials and tribulations of our lives don't accurately reflect who we are and the greatness we are ultimately capable of.

In his youth, Einstein experienced significant developmental and behavioural challenges, yet he was able to overcome the immense challenges and pain of his past and achieve extraordinary personal greatness in later years.

Albert Einstein was born in Germany in 1879 to upper-middle-class parents. Despite his later accomplishments, his formative years showed nothing of the brilliance that was to follow in adulthood. At the age of three, while other children were asking questions that involved the basic "who", "why", "where" and "what", and being understood (most of the time), Einstein's world was silent as he was unable to speak. Much to his family's relief, by the time he was four years old he did discover language, but he was not able to communicate easily or effectively, let alone use sentences containing four or more words, talk about his day or answer basic questions typical of children his age. In fact, his speech and communication challenges were so pronounced that many in his immediate family circle believed that he was developmentally and cognitively impaired.

While Albert was clashing with the outside world, at the same time he was on a self-designated life mission. This mission was fuelled by the gift of a magnetometer, a compass, given to him at the time. Einstein marvelled at the mysterious powers that guided the metal needle on the compass and committed himself to better understand the unseen forces involved in moving the dial. At around the same time, he started taking violin lessons and fortunately he fell deeply in love with music. This was a fortuitous event as music training, both as a child and in adulthood, is associated with improvements in IQ, mathematical abilities and overall cognitive flexibility.[2] Moreover, music offered Einstein an escape from the challenges and struggles of his world, albeit a temporary one.

As he grew up, his immediate and extended family members became reconciled to his limitations and labelled him as a "simple" child who was "backward", thereby absolving any expectations of him attaining "normality" in his lifetime.

Not being able to verbally communicate well negatively impacted on Einstein's self-confidence, self-esteem and self-worth. Determined to improve his speech, Einstein ingeniously developed a unique strategy to converse, which involved practising sentences quietly to himself before speaking to those around him.

Albert's impediment opened the floodgates of teasing, ridicule and social isolation. His defensive response was one of anger, rebelliousness, total disdain for authority and an aversion to any form of conformity. According to Einstein, "unthinking respect for authority is the greatest enemy of the truth." By the time he reached primary school, he was nothing short of a handful.

Now labelled and defined by his behavioural, learning and language difficulties, some of his teachers made a point of expressing their views that he would not amount to anything in life, stripping him of a sense of personal value and greater purpose in the world. This negative narrative is not easy for a self-confident adult to process, let alone a vulnerable child. With his confidence further eroded, Einstein's speech impairment developed into echolalia, a condition where a person meaninglessly repeats sentences and other people's words.

For many children (and adults), being different equates to being excluded and for Albert this was a distressing and perpetual reality. Not able to play games or engage in age-appropriate social activities with other children, Einstein compensated by creating an imaginary parallel universe of his own, frequented by long bouts of daydreaming. Puzzles also helped him fill the social vacuum he existed in.

As the years passed, Albert continued to struggle with verbal communication and combined with social isolation, loneliness, ridicule and mockery culminated in an explosive temper further alienating him from the world around him.

Yet despite all these compounded challenges (and possibly *because* of them) Einstein was able to develop many strong character traits and skills that would serve him well later in life, including unwavering determination, tenaciousness, grit and persistence.

Albert's personal challenges were magnified by his Jewish ethnicity and being subjected to aggressive anti-Semitism. His cultural and religious differences resulted in harassment, frequent beatings and further isolation both at school and outside of it. It is impossible to imagine how vulnerable, lonely, isolated and scared Einstein must have felt during those formative years, which are supposed to be carefree and filled with joy and laughter.

Occupational and speech therapists explain that a speech disorder follows someone throughout the course of their life and this was certainly the case for Einstein. By the age of nine, he was not only battling with verbal communication, but also reading, basic comprehension and memory pertaining to language.

Notwithstanding, Albert was able to effectively compensate if not altogether overcome these learning barriers in his chosen areas of interest (science and physics) by using pictures and images as opposed to letters, words and vocabulary.

As the years passed, typical play, playmates and sports participation were still a rarity, leaving Einstein little choice but to sit alone with his questions about the world and the universe as a whole. The net effect of his solitude was the continued development and growth of his powerful imagination which he started to use to formulate an expansive life and perceivably far-fetched theories.

The weight of difference and perpetual struggle continued to fuel Einstein's anger issues and feelings of resentment, culminating in an overt repulsion to all forms of dogma and authority.

Despite the hardships that were taking place in Albert's life, there was one safe space that was a constant and that was his family and home environment. Although there are no indications that it was an overly warm, supportive or loving environment, it did seem to provide Einstein with a sanctuary — a safe space where he felt some degree of certainty, consistency and familiarity. Sadly, this too would unravel for Albert.

As a teenager, the family business collapsed under the pressure of the recession and unfavourable market forces at the time. In an attempt to get back on their feet, Einstein's parents and siblings were forced to move to Italy. They made the decision to leave Albert in Germany with distant relatives so that he could complete his schooling. The pressure was all too much: his language and learning difficulties, an intense hatred for conformity and the rigidity of the German schooling system at the time, anti-Semitism, social isolation and an absent family unit resulted in Einstein having an emotional breakdown and falling into a deep depression.

He was forced to drop out of school (although it was never established whether he was asked to leave or left of his own accord) and joined his family in Pavia, Italy. Unable to reconcile, let alone accept that their son was a 15-year-old high-school dropout, Einstein's family insisted that he continued with his education. The goal was for him to enrol in a technical college located in Zurich, Switzerland. But because he hadn't completed high school and was at least two years younger than the average applicant, he would require a substantial concession to attend. Undeterred and optimistic, Albert studied tirelessly in order to meet the basic entrance exam requirements.

Later that year, based on the incredible promise he had shown in the area of physics, and a letter to the director of the college from a respected and influential family friend, Albert was given the opportunity to take the entrance exam. He failed horribly, but did excel in the subjects he was passionate about, such as maths and science. But in the other subjects, including literature, politics, botany and zoology, he fared poorly.

However, seeing Albert's untapped potential in physics, the college director suggested that Albert complete another year of high school and recommended that he stay in Switzerland and attend the cantonal school, which was located approximately 50 kilometres away from the college. Eager to do whatever was necessary to be accepted into the college, Einstein and his family took the director's advice. The teaching philosophy of the cantonal school was unique and progressive for the time and as such was based on ideas formulated by a renowned educational reformer, Johann Pestalozzi. The teachers encouraged the students to use imagery in their learning process and believed strongly in nurturing individuality and the inner dignity of a child. This aligned perfectly with Einstein's personality, learning style and expectations of education. Rote drills, memorisation and force-fed facts were replaced by observation, intuition, conceptual thinking and visualisation, all areas that Einstein excelled in.

Albert loved attending the school and especially its learning methodology, a far cry from the rigid authoritarian and conformist models of his difficult and painful past in Germany.

Another very important change took place in Albert's life while attending school in Switzerland. He boarded with a large, warm and embracing family, who welcomed him and provided an environment of genuine care and safety. The family was non-conformist, non-judgemental and all accepting. It was almost as if Albert was given the opportunity to rewrite his personal script. Who he was, where he came from and the internal struggles he had faced his entire life were inconsequential in his new home. The spotlight was on who he was and what he wanted to become.

Moreover, Jost Winteler, the family patriarch and a teacher at Albert's new school, shared Albert's aversion to German militarism and nationalism in general. Jost was approachable, honest and idealistic and helped

Einstein shape his social philosophies for the future, including pacifism, democratic socialism, individual liberty and freedom of expression. Albert finally felt accepted and loved for who he was, rather than being critically evaluated for what he was lacking. In this environment, his psychological defences and emotional walls receded, and he displayed a charisma, wit and humour never seen before.

The combination of support and autonomy resulted in a new reality for Albert where he was able to blossom and flourish. There were gaping holes in key subjects at school like chemistry and languages that required major remedial work and additional lessons, but in the areas where his passions lay (science, maths and music), he excelled. In a letter Jost wrote to Einstein's family, he notes, "but with Albert I got used to finding mediocre grades along with very good ones, and I am therefore not disconsolate about them."[3]

When the school year came to an end, Einstein managed to score the second highest overall grade in the class. For a former "dropout", this was unprecedented. Ready to tackle the next leg of his formal education, he took the entrance exam, which included written and oral sections, for the Zurich Polytechnic. Of the nine students who took the entrance exam, Albert achieved the highest grade and was accepted.

As they say, the rest is history, as Albert Einstein went on to become one of the most influential scientific thinkers of all time. His achievements include the quantum theory of light, the general theory of relativity, the special theory of relativity, the photoelectric effect and the wave particle effect. He won the Nobel Prize for physics in 1921 and was chosen as the most influential person of the 20th century by *Time* magazine.

Einstein's story is one of exceptional resilience. His life's journey reveals that tremendous gifts and many abilities are acquired from enduring the struggle itself. For Einstein, it was a clear visual understanding of certain concepts, persistence, determination, adaptability, divergent thinking, imagination and unwavering passion for what he loved, but equally importantly it highlighted the critical importance of the influence of the people who share our lives and our environment in shaping and enabling our future reality.

Like Einstein, many of us have experienced adversity, whether in the form of abuse (physical or psychological or both), neglect, poverty or health impediments (cognitive, behavioural or physical). What his story teaches us is that we are not defined by where we come from, how we were brought up or even by our genetically inherited abilities. While there is an undeniable influence, we are greater than each part, or even the collective sum of them all. At some point in our lives we will all have a choice. The choice to live the life we want to and let go of the self-imposed barriers, towering emotional walls, impenetrable defences and fears, or continue to be imprisoned by them. Like all accomplishments, whether in sport, music, art, sciences or business, this requires commitment to the process, training and guidance, repetition, persistence, refinement and an acceptance that we will fail along the way.

If we explore the lives of some of the great classical composers, it is clear that they too had to make these kinds of choices. The author Adam Grant poignantly points out in his 2017 book, *Originals: How Non-conformists Move the World*, that success in any endeavour equates to effort,[4] and he uses the great classical composers as an example. According to Grant, music aficionados generally agree that the musical genius Mozart composed six extraordinary pieces. What is less well known is that he composed another 600 works during that process. Another iconic composer, Johann Sebastian Bach, produced three critically outstanding works, but in his musical journey he composed more than 1,000 pieces.

Success in creating the life you have always wished for is commensurate with the work that you willing to put in.

Resilience is not something you are either born with or not; it is a personal journey that requires courage. The courage to move forward, the courage to face and move past our fears and self-limiting behaviours and the courage to decide on what we want for our lives.

WHAT IS RESILIENCE?

Since the onset of the COVID-19 pandemic, resilience has become one of the most popular concepts for teams and businesses to focus on, and it would be difficult to find a team or business that doesn't have the word "resilience" as part of its core value set. This is not surprising considering that COVID-19 has been superimposed on the Fourth Industrial Revolution (4IR), creating a new set of socio-political-economic conditions, the likes of which the world has never seen.

> Fixed behaviours, no matter how effective they are, cannot defend against the major changes we are experiencing within the world today.

It is as if the world we live in and share has become scorched, not only by drought or through the compounded effects of decades of global warming, but by negative human emotions of fear, uncertainty and panic.

Our historical understanding of resilience has been centred around grit, greater resolve, more persistence, the ability to "pivot" and unwavering determination in every and all endeavours. While these are powerful psychosocial traits and are key contributors to human performance and success, they are limited within the context of the promotion of long-term resilience.

The reason for this is that a new set of socio-economic conditions emerged seemingly overnight and continue to rapidly and exponentially evolve, morph and recalibrate. Fixed behaviours, no matter how powerful, cannot defend against the changes that we are experiencing and are likely to go through in the future.

If resilience is broader and more expansive than persistence, determination or grit, then what is it? The *Oxford English Dictionary* defines resilience as:

> *noun:* capacity to recover quickly from difficulties; toughness

While the definition of resilience is clean, simple and easy to grasp, there are two significant limitations within this description. The first lies with the notion of simply "recovering" from life's challenges. While recovery is advantageous in all areas of health and wellbeing, it is a reactive situation that doesn't necessarily prepare us for impending and ongoing challenges. In many respects, it locks us into the past as opposed to creating a stage for improved coping and performance in an uncertain future.

The second issue with the definition has to do with the broader concept of toughness, either mental or physical, and its relationship with overcoming challenges, adversity, change and uncertainty.

IS MENTAL TOUGHNESS AND GRIT ENOUGH?

In 2007 I was offered my dream job – a senior director with the Chinese Olympic team, which had a real shot at winning the games and making sporting history. I committed myself to making a difference, ready to throw everything I had and more into this once-in-a-lifetime role. It was a moment of clarity where every athlete I had ever worked with, every book and research paper I had ever read, every weekend and holiday I had ever worked through had culminated in this incredible opportunity.

Within days of my arrival in Beijing, I realised the sheer scale and magnitude of the position I had been given and the immense challenges that came with it. The phrase "Careful what you wish for" couldn't have been more apt.

Essentially, I was an outsider going into an established and well-oiled team. The athletes had lived, trained, eaten and socialised with each other for years, if not decades. They were a tight-knit family who were suspicious and guarded when it came to foreigners. Being accepted, trusted and respected was going to take time and a lot of effort on my part and, even then, it wasn't a given.

At the same time, the expectations from the administrators, coaches and stakeholders (in this case, the Chinese government) were stratospheric. The weeks and weekends were undifferentiated and the nights and days became merged. In other words, each day was nothing short of a marathon. Support in any form was a rarity, which paralleled the complete social isolation I was experiencing due to the language barrier, movement restrictions (not being allowed to leave the training precinct), and limited internet access and phone services. To add pressure to a strained situation, the leaders and administrators showed little to no transparency, care, respect, clarity or appreciation – in other words, justice and fairness in all its forms was scarce. Lastly, the authority or control to make decisions pertaining to my professional responsibilities, let alone personal decisions as to when I exercised, when to wake up and when I went to sleep, were removed until further notice.

It was a tough environment, but what I had taken to Beijing was mental toughness, grit, hardiness, resolve, determination and strength of will forged in an abundance of childhood adversity and refined during compulsory military training, all things that I believed would stand me in good stead – but I was wrong.

As the weeks passed, my dream job turned into a nightmare experience and took a huge toll on me. At first it manifested in a higher frequency of colds and flu that I put down to the notoriously high levels of pollution in the city. But I then began to lose mental clarity, focus, motivation and the ability to learn quickly and progressively. Finally, there was an emotional cost. My low mood progressed into states of mild depression and anxiety, specifically in the form of obsessive-compulsive disorder (OCD), most notably a need for symmetry and orderliness.

I kept telling myself that I had been through challenges before and could draw on resources and skills I had developed and mastered historically to overcome this. I self-dialogued, telling myself, "You've got this"; I tried to exercise as regularly as possible, avoided alcohol and limited coffee to half a cup in the morning. But none of this was enough and, in fact, didn't even touch the sides.

The steady decline in my health forced me to shift my goal orientation away from medium- and long-term aspirations to very short-term ambitions, which turned out to be simply getting through the day. I was perplexed. How was this even possible? I had been through some really difficult situations in my life, yet this challenge impacted me differently and so broadly, causing a radical decline in my emotional, mental and physical wellbeing. The resilience tactics I had polished and refined over decades of struggle seemed to be rendered utterly ineffective in this situation. Even with all the grit and determination and persistence, I ended up as one of the 34.3 per cent[5] of individuals who become significantly impacted by adversity.

Perhaps I was being too hard on myself, after all many of the stressors I was experiencing were established triggers in mental and physical health compromise. For example, long working hours and high demands increase the risk of developing anxiety, depression or sleep disorders by 60 per cent, a lack of support by 38 per cent, not feeling valued or having limited growth opportunities by 49 per cent and not having a say or control in matters that directly affect you on a daily basis by 42 per cent.[6] Independently, these stressors can have a profound impact on mental health, yet I was experiencing them collectively. In hindsight, it is little wonder that I was hanging on by a thread.

After several long and incredibly challenging months, the opportunity arose for me to travel to England with the Chinese national tennis team. Five extremely talented women, some of whom would achieve rankings as high as number 1 and 2 in the world, were on their way to Wimbledon (the most prestigious event on the tennis calendar) and due to my extensive experience in the sport, having worked with many of the world's best players and teams since 2002, I was instructed to accompany them.

WIMBLEDON – THE GRASS BECOMES GREENER

Being back in the familiar world of tennis validated the stress of my work environment in Beijing and the perceived weight of my challenges. The excitement and bustle of Wimbledon, reconnecting with friends and a more manageable schedule transformed my physical and emotional wellbeing within days. I was once again training hard and felt energised, motivated, passionate, focused and excited about life. For three weeks, it felt like a psychological load had been lifted, liberating the best version of myself. But the tournament was nearing completion, meaning I would soon have to return to Beijing and my perceived challenges. This realisation triggered many negative emotions as I relived many of my bad experiences.

During the final week of the event, I was fortunate to receive an impromptu and unexpected coaching session on reframing by the iconic Billy Jean King. "Reframing" is another term used to describe cognitive reappraisal, the ability to screen and evaluate our thoughts and replace negative ones with positive ones. It involves conscious reassessment or reinterpretation of adversity to find a positive perspective and something meaningful through the challenging events of one's life. Positive reframing has been shown to be a strong predictor of resilience, especially in adolescents and athletes.[7]

I first met Billy Jean King in 2003 when I worked with Martina Navratilova at Wimbledon, helping her to overcome a chronic foot injury. Martina was one of my first big international tennis clients. Fast-forward five years and I was back in SW19, although under very different circumstances. Late one evening in the Wimbledon gym, Billy Jean was cycling on the stationary bike next to mine. We started talking and at first it was about the tournament and the results thereof, but I soon found myself describing my time in Beijing and how its challenges had impacted me so profoundly.

She graciously listened for a few minutes before offering me some advice that turned out to be central in me making a significant life change and which was related to the promotion of future resilience. The first pearl of wisdom she imparted was that pressure is a privilege. She expounded on this by saying that anyone who finds themselves in an environment where they are exposed to high expectations, coupled with extraordinary demands, has to have some degree of inherent ability, skill and industry recognition. This strongly resonated with me, but it wasn't the psychological turning point. It was her next statement that has stayed with me since that evening chat in June 2008. She looked at me, stopped cycling and said, "Remember this, Richard, all champions adapt."

I wanted to prove myself and be a "champion" in my own capacity and role within the team, but I realised I was holding onto old skills, values and beliefs and I had failed to grow, to evolve and subsequently to cope.

While I did feel better (at least momentarily) from the conversation we'd had, it took a few days for what Billy Jean had said to me to really infuse itself into my consciousness. I started thinking about all the coaches, athletes, doctors, trainers and physical therapists I had studied and worked with over the duration of my career and how they would respond to the opportunity I had been given. After almost eight months of viewing the glass half empty due to unmanaged stress and pressure, I had finally grasped the magnitude of my role. To hold any position within such an accomplished team of athletes and coaches wasn't merely a privilege but an opportunity unlikely to be repeated, and I had to appreciate and value each and every precious moment.

PRESSURE IS A PRIVILEGE

The realisation of the uniqueness of my situation, amidst the further upcoming challenges I would be facing, was not something I was going to let fade. "This is your once-in-a-lifetime opportunity" is a phrase I reminded myself of every day. This repeated reminder of how pressure is a privilege jump-started my motivation, drive and passion. My passion was ignited but more importantly I was smiling. Reflecting back on the experience, I realise that nothing had changed for me on an external level; the shift was entirely from within. It was the idea that "champions adapt" that was to have the greatest influence on my future within the team and beyond. Upon reflection (and a very deep dive, at that) I realised that up until this point, I had been rigid and admittedly stagnant, employing protocols that had worked for other teams and individuals with vastly different needs and circumstances.

The issue that was negatively impacting my health and performance stemmed from an inability to adapt. I knew I needed to change, although I didn't know how or what steps to take to make this a reality. Within the context of resilience, I had already **Pressure is a privilege.** taken a giant leap. Unbeknown to me at the time, the belief that "pressure is a privilege" is fundamentally the expression of cognitive reappraisal – one of the most influential of all resilience skills. Altering the team dynamic by increasing support and strengthening relationships would be the next step in my resilience journey.

This required that I meaningfully connect to the team and all its members, but the barrier to this was undeniably the language. This was my call to action and so I made a decision to learn Mandarin (or at the very least, try). The challenge was that I was so self-reliant that it made it difficult for me to ask for help. **Champions adapt.** But as hard as it was for me to reach out to others, I stretched myself and asked some of the respected and influential members of the team for help. While they had always been quite distant towards me, to my surprise they enthusiastically agreed.

To be frank, I was a terrible student and struggled with the tones of the language, which I couldn't seem to recognise. Mandarin uses four primary tones to differentiate meaning and, because of my struggles, I was a source of much laughter and entertainment to most of the team as I sounded like a 15-year-old poodle! It was horrible, but the embarrassment was worth it as it broke the ice and brought down the defensive walls on both sides.

I continued to immerse myself in the language and the rich culture, but more importantly in the lives of the people I was there to help. I created a new template for myself for how I worked and lived that was completely malleable and dynamic and different from any other way I had worked before. Equipped with a few phrases and words (although no one really ever did understand me), I felt comfortable enough to explore the city on my own (when allowed to leave the training facility). Within weeks, my health had radically improved from what I believe was increased social support, the newfound skill of cognitive reappraisal, greater optimism, more openness and the continual acquisition of new psychological skills, such as proactivity and extroversion, which I learnt from the athletes themselves.

Essentially, the armoury I had developed through all my struggles in childhood and early adulthood, from the neglect, abuse and uncertainty I faced, was completely obsolete in my current circumstances. Resilience was no longer confined to toughness, intensity and pushing through no matter the cost. And I saw it clearly for the first time.

> Resilience is the ability to emotionally, mentally and physically adapt to stress, challenge, adversity and change.

REAL-TIME ADAPTABILITY

My experience in Beijing illustrates that adaptability is possible within the medium or long term but it is important to consider that the ability to adapt in real-time is equally (if not more) important in the promotion of resilience. This is a skill that takes much effort and practice to master.

The individual rhythmic gymnastics final at the Tokyo Olympics in 2021 epitomises instantaneous adaptability and cognitive flexibility at the highest level and demonstrates its transformative potential under some of the most difficult and challenging circumstances.

To provide some perspective to this Olympic event, for 21 years Russia reigned supreme on the mat. Women's individual all-round rhythmic gymnastics had become synonymous with one story and a predictable ending. Would the Tokyo Olympics be any different? If so, the competitor would be facing a formidable pair of Russian twins, Dina and Arina Averina. With a track record of a collective total of 62 gold medals from the major lead-up events to Tokyo, including the World Championships, the European Championships, the World Cup Final, World Games and Grand Prix Final, the twins were practically unbeatable.

In a strong pack of gymnasts, one contender immediately stood out from the rest. Israeli gymnast Linoy Ashram was in incredible form, fiercely competitive and highly motivated. Despite winning a handful of medals since 1952, Israel as a nation had never won a medal in rhythmic gymnastics before.

The stage was set for one of the most captivating battles in the history of the sport. Rhythmic gymnasts are scored on the artistry of their performances set to music and the skill with which they execute difficult manoeuvres using the handheld apparatuses. These apparatuses include a hoop, ball, pair of clubs and ribbons and each athlete has 75–90 seconds to complete an action-packed routine to "wow" the judges and audiences alike.

Ten finalists competed on the 13m x 13m mat for the prized gold medal. All the routines and performances proved exceptional, but it was the colossal battle between two athletes, Linoy Ashram and Dina Averina, that captivated the audience and the judges.

In the first event, the hoop, Ashram narrowly took the lead, with a score of 27.550 over Averina's 27.200. The stadium erupted (despite there only being a handful of coaches, medical staff, family and team members in the audience due to COVID-19 restrictions) and the Israeli support team appeared to be hyperventilating with joy. Watching at home, my wife and I were standing on the couch, cheering with our arms in the air.

The second event was the ball, and both gymnasts mesmerised the audience and judges with their poise, grace and incredible athleticism and they tied with a score of 28.300. While Ashram was still in the lead, it was by a narrow margin going into the third apparatus – the clubs. This rivalry was undoubtedly bringing out the best in these two athletes. Ashram won the rotation, scoring an astonishing 28.650 over Averina's 28.150. The tension continued to grow as all eyes were focused on the engrossing contest between the gymnasts. My palms were sweaty, my breathing rapid and my heart was pounding. I felt like I was in that arena, not 14,000 kilometres away.

One more event to go – the ribbon – for a possible history-defining moment for the Israeli.

At .850 points ahead, Ashram needed a solid performance, with a good mix of skill, execution and creativity. She stepped onto the mat, performed her routine hand taps on her thighs and threw herself into her final routine. She delivered with the precision and energy of the previous apparatus, but somehow, mid-routine, she dropped the ribbon. The crowd and undoubtedly millions of viewers around the world held their breath and covered their faces with their hands. I was lying on the floor, my hands covering my face, repeatedly exclaiming, "No, no, no!"

The cost of Ashram's momentary lapse would be a minimum of .30 points and it might just have cost her the gold. Incredibly, in one of the greatest displays of real-time adaptability, Ashram effortlessly picked up the ribbon and decided to increase the complexity of her already difficult routine in order to claw back points. The commentators were astounded and repeatedly referenced this dynamic routine recalibration. Facing an error or failure of this magnitude in any area of our lives, many, if not most of us, would simply want to finish our metaphorical routine and hope for the best while we regroup and fixate on the past failures.

Not Linoy. It was probably the most remarkable display of control, beauty and athleticism I have ever seen – but was it enough? Was adapting her routine the right decision?

Averina stepped forward for her final routine with a small, confident smile on her face. I had seen that look many times during my 20-year sports career and it was the surety of impending success. As I anticipated, her routine was flawless, not surprising as the world's top-ranked rhythmic gymnast. The judges and crowd agreed.

Averina's routine was the last of the tournament, and with it the most nail-biting rhythmic gymnastics event in decades was concluded. To prevent even the slightest margin of error or controversy, the judges spent what seemed like hours deliberating the final score. Who would be crowned the champion of Tokyo and the 32nd Olympic Games? Finally the official results were in. While Dina Averina had scored the highest in the ribbon with a strong 24.00 points, Ashram's adapted routine scored 23.300, proving to be enough to give her a strong .150-point overall lead in the four rotations. She was the champion and first medal holder for Israel in the sport of rhythmic gymnastics and the first gold medal ever won by a female athlete from the small Middle East nation.

The lesson in all this is that if Ashram had continued her routine without adaptation, the final outcome would have been very different. It is also a message of the power of self-belief and not allowing setbacks, however large or small they may seem, to bring you down or hold you back from your dreams.

I learnt a saying during my first visit to Moscow back in 2005 that has always resonated with me, "nevozmozhnoye vozmozhno" – the impossible is possible. In this instance, it was a highly adaptable Israeli athlete reminding her Russian counterpart of this powerful message.

PART 2

THE NEUROSCIENCE
OF RESILIENCE

EIGHT POWERFUL LESSONS

Human resilience has been a topic of significant interest since the early 1970s and has been extensively researched in a variety of populations, and in many different contexts, providing a wealth of knowledge that we can use to apply to our own lives and unique challenges. The scientific exploration that began many decades ago was principally in the area of childhood adversity and development. Since childhood adversity is not a choice and requires exceptional resources to overcome, it is an important departure point for the next section of the book. Moreover, there is an incredible depth of knowledge and understanding in this area that continues to grow on a daily basis.

This part of the book will provide you with deep insights, together with a plethora of skills that will not only support you in developing your personal resilience but will also ultimately promote success in many areas of your life, whether it be professional, in a sport or in your relationships.

Decades of research has culminated in eight core resilience lessons that look at the impact of our childhood in shaping response to stress, how our intrinsic personality influences coping mechanisms, the importance of further developing and refining existing resilience competencies, new skill acquisition, and most notably, the importance of health promotion. Together, these attributes have the potential to support our greatest dreams, hopes and aspirations, provided they form a basis from which we perceive and react to our challenges, difficulties, failures, setbacks and painful experiences.

One of the strongest research articles in the area of childhood resilience and future potential was a 2019 review published in *Translational Psychiatry*.[1] The Australian research team, headed by Gin Malhi, was able to capture a range of key resilience theories and concepts and skilfully link them to genetic, neurobiological, psychological, behavioural and social factors. Many of the profound life lessons outlined in the pages that follow draw inspiration from this paper and research articles like it.

LESSON 1

OUR PERSONALITY SUPPORTS RESILIENCE

Even though adaptability and cognitive flexibility best describe resilience, the reality is that resilience is by no means limited to a single trait or behaviour. Rather, resilience is complex and layered and has strong associations with a person's individual personality and genetic make-up.

While our personality and genetics strongly shape the way we perceive, relate to and engage with the outside world, it is both their independent and combined influence on how we react to and respond to stress (i.e. the activation and inhibition of the stress axis) that ultimately determines a trajectory either towards increasing health compromise (when we can't manage these responses) or towards the development of successful adaptation (when we can).

■

THE BIG FIVE

Almost five decades of research has revealed a group of personality traits that positively influence the way we respond to negative life experiences. These qualities have been shown to not only offer protection from adversity, challenge and emotional hurt, but also have the potential to enhance and shape our future reality. These core qualities include extroversion, openness, agreeableness, conscientiousness and emotional stability.

A large 2018 meta-analysis done by researchers from Japan, the US and Canada, involving 30 studies and including 15,609 individuals (both adults and children), found significantly higher levels of resilience in those who were more extroverted, open, agreeable and conscientious.[1] The review showed that these traits can support resilience, whether in isolation or in combination, with the greatest positive influence coming from either extroversion or conscientiousness. In many respects this makes sense in that when facing challenges and/or adversity, by being more extroverted it creates greater opportunities for social support, while conscientiousness will steer us in the direction of order, structure and goal orientation, mitigating the experience of overwhelm and a lack of control.

The Big Five

At the same time, those individuals who demonstrated a tendency towards anxiety, negativity and self-doubt (i.e. neurosis) were less resilient and more emotionally and mentally vulnerable in response to demanding and stressful events.

By supporting our capacity to rapidly adapt to novel and unpredictable situations, and due to their significant influence on the promotion and expression of social confidence, perceptiveness, originality and sensibility, these personality traits are commonly referred to as the "Big Five'.

At this point you might be thinking, "But what if I don't possess one or more of these traits? Does this mean that I'm not resilient?" The truth is that we are all able to develop and grow these characteristics should we choose to. This brings resilience well within the reach of all of us, no matter where you are in your life and what you may be facing at any given time.

Before discussing and exploring the different ways we are able to positively influence the "Big Five" personality traits, it is important to

Personality quick assessment

I see myself as: I see myself as:

Closed to new ideas	**Openness**	Enjoying new experiences
Predictable and patterned		Curious
Resistant to change	1 2 3 4 5 6 7 8 9 10	Unconventional/unorthodox
Conservative		Imaginative

Impulsive and unreliable	**Conscientious**	Self-disciplined
Disorganised		Generally organised
A procrastinator	1 2 3 4 5 6 7 8 9 10	Goal-orientated
Reactive and unmeasured		Responsible and accountable

Quiet and reflective	**Extroversion**	Sociable
Reserved		Enjoys the limelight
Self-conscious	1 2 3 4 5 6 7 8 9 10	Outgoing
Uncomfortable being the centre of attention		Warm

A bit anxious	**Emotional stability**	Calm
Irritable		Fairly confident
Stressed	1 2 3 4 5 6 7 8 9 10	Emotionally stable (most of the time)
Up and down emotionally		Adaptable

Sceptical	**Agreeable**	Forgiving
Demanding		Modest
Stubborn	1 2 3 4 5 6 7 8 9 10	Empathetic
A little insensitive		Altruistic

consider that they exist on a continuum and are not delineated by a simple "I am" or "I am not" in a specific area.

The quick assessment on page 37 will help you to identify your key strengths and vulnerabilities within this set as well as establish future directions for growth and self-improvement. My suggestion is that you perform the test with a close friend, family member or partner. In this way, we can overcome our tendency to see what we want to, as opposed to seeing what we need to.

Circle the number that best describes where you feel your level of personality trait falls on the line. Following this, ask your partner to rate you objectively. Somewhere in the middle you will find clarity.

The beauty of this basic test is its simplicity and transparency.

Being one step ahead of cognitive bias

During a recent call with Craig, a very close friend, he described some of the challenges he was facing at work and the distress it was causing him. He worked for a multinational company, where the professional environment was centred on a command-and-control style and allowed for very little autonomy, flexibility, creativity or personal expression. At the same time, there was tremendous infighting in the organisation and internal politics as power struggles existed within the leadership group. Appreciation and growth opportunities were rare, creating a very oppressive and joyless environment. But Craig was paid very well, had a large family and many financial obligations and as a consequence was unable (or unwilling) to resign and find a healthier professional environment. His only option was to develop his personal resilience and try to equip himself better to handle the relentless challenges and pressures he was facing.

I asked Craig his perceptions of his own personality. "Are you open?" I asked. "Very much so," he replied. I continued, "Do you see yourself as conscientious, agreeable, extroverted and emotionally grounded?" Craig responded affirmatively to conscientious and agreeable and no to extroverted and emotionally grounded.

We then did the simple assessment together, viewing these traits in their totality and as a continuum rather than definitive yes or no. To his surprise, Craig scored low on openness, high for conscientiousness, high for extroversion, low for emotional stability and fared moderately on agreeableness.

The objectivity in his self-evaluation gave Craig the core focus areas that he needed to develop in order to build and grow his resilience. These areas related to his openness and emotional stability.

Craig's resilience plan would centre on four behaviours:

1. Regular (daily) aerobic exercise in order to support dopamine (the molecule that drives openness and creativity), BDNF (brain-derived neutrophic factor, which supports emotional stability and cognitive potential) and serotonin (which influences emotional behaviours and cognitive flexibility)
2. Improved stress management with 10–15 minutes of daily meditation, deep breathing or yoga
3. The decision to consciously look at daily issues and challenges and to ask himself, "How can I approach this differently?"
4. A commitment to be more persistent in difficult endeavours.

Personality and brain chemistry

Because genetics and neurochemistry have such a profound effect on human potential, it should come as no surprise that the Big Five traits are strongly influenced by these factors. The most influential neurochemicals in the positive expression of a resilient personality include dopamine and norepinephrine (specifically pertaining to extroversion, openness, conscientiousness and agreeableness), oxytocin (contributes strongly to

Primary neurochemical influence in Big Five personality traits

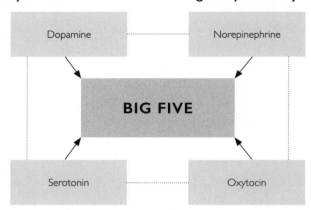

extroversion and conscientiousness and protects against neuroticism) as well as serotonin (supports emotional regulation and openness).

While the role of oxytocin and serotonin is significant, the headline story from a Big Five personality perspective is dopamine and norepinephrine.

Dopamine and norepinephrine have a remarkably synergistic relationship that can bridge the divide between curiosity and self-discipline, imagination and goal orientation as well as confidence and modesty. When the expression, transport, signalling and metabolism of these neurochemicals are in an ideal balance (not too much or too little), resilience flourishes and our personality shines brightly, especially in those moments of challenge and adversity.

One of the more significant influences in supporting and maintaining ideal dopamine and norepinephrine levels and balance are two enzymes: catechol-O-methyltransferase (COMT) and dopamine beta-hydroxylase (DBH).

DBH is an enzyme responsible for converting dopamine into norepinephrine, a neurochemical that has many resilience influences that go beyond our personality traits. Some of these include protection against anxiety, improved focus, concentration, perserverence and the modulation of blood sugar levels. COMT is one of several enzymes that inactivates the neurochemicals dopamine, norepinephrine and epinephrine, ensuring an optimal balance within the brain based on the demands of a given situation. This delicate balance ultimately impacts adaptability, mood stability and cognitive function, together with many aspects of our personality.

It is important to bear in mind that a fundamental resilience principle, and in many respects a central premise of this book, is that our neurochemistry underpins many of our actions. At the same time, this relationship is bidirectional (i.e. our behaviour also determines and influences our neurochemistry). Knowing this, an important accompaniment to skill development and acquisition (such as seeing the benefit of adversity, the regulation of our emotions, etc.) is the deliberate promotion and regulation of neurochemical balance. In the case of cultivating the Big Five personality traits, this means supporting and balancing COMT, due to its role in dopamine and norepinephrine metabolism.

A good starting point would be to ensure a rich supply of B vitamins, specifically B2, B6, B9, B12, and vitamin D, together with magnesium from either food or supplemented sources, as these nutrients are necessary for this enzyme production within the body.

Nowhere is the individuality and uniqueness of the human condition more obvious than in the expression behaviours of the COMT enzyme. Genetic studies have shown that individuals can inherit a mutation that either radically increases expression or decreases its production by 300–400 per cent.[2]

The consequence of this can be chronically raised or, alternatively, reduced levels of dopamine, norepinephrine and epinephrine, which in turn impact our ability to effectively cope with stress and pressure and adversely affects many facets of our personality by making us less confident, more insular and closed. This highlights the value in performing personalised genetic testing in your resilience journey as well as the fundamental importance of conscious awareness of all things that influence COMT expression.

The environment and personality – worlds colliding

The influence of our physical environment on our personality is seldom considered. By environment, I am specifically referring to cosmetics, household cleaning products, food containers, processed foods, environmental chemicals, heavy metals, as well as air and water quality. These factors should be taken into account because they are saturated with xenoestrogens and other potentially damaging composites. Xenoestrogens are compounds that imitate the hormone oestrogen, which can be natural or synthetic in origin.

Common xenoestrogens

Compound	Management strategy
Pesticides and herbicides	Try to select organic fruits and vegetables if/where available. Alternatively, wash your produce more carefully.
Polychlorinated biphenyls	Limit animal fat in your diet. This includes butter, cheese, cream, poultry and meat.
Bisphenol A (BPA) and phthalate esters	Limit your exposure to plastics as much as possible. Replace plastic containers and products with glass, stainless steel and other natural products.
Alkylphenols	Try to choose natural detergents and personal care products. Natural and non-toxic options are freely available at health stores and large supermarkets.
Alkyl esters of p-hydroxybenzoic acid (parabens)	Avoid food preservatives and try to use natural personal care products where possible.
Metalloestrogens: aluminium, cadmium	Avoid exposure to cigarette smoke and personal care products that contain aluminium, specifically deodorants and antiperspirants.
Synthetic progestins and oestrogens	These compounds are found in fertility treatments, the contraceptive pill, hormone replacement therapy and some personal care products. Avoidance may not always be possible. If you are taking any of these medications, speak to your doctor about lifestyle changes that may offer similar support.

In many respects, the connecting thread between our personality and the physical world is COMT. Not only does COMT play a major role in the metabolism of dopamine and norepinephrine, it is also important in the breaking down of toxic xenoestrogens and overall elimination from our bodies.[3] Considering that COMT production is tightly governed (i.e. finite) and bound to genetic inheritance, chronic exposure to xenoestrogens may adversely affect stress hormone metabolism together with immune system behaviours, resulting in disproportionate and sustained stress responses and greater emotional vulnerability.

In order to better support the development and/or refinement of the Big Five personality traits by optimising dopamine and norepinephrine metabolism, it would be advantageous to become more aware and selective of our physical environment, especially for those who underexpress the enzyme (due to an genetic variant known as COMT AA, which is associated with a significant reduction in COMT enzyme expression) and who are prone to anxiety and feel overwhelmed when confronted with stressful events.

To navigate this complex topic, I have compiled the table on p.42 to highlight some of the more common xenoestrogens we are exposed to on a day-to-day basis and ways we can reduce this burden, thereby protecting our bodies and minds.[4]

■

PLUS ONE – OPTIMISM

Optimism reflects the extent to which you believe your future is going to be positive. For years, the relationship between optimism and resilience has been a key area of research. For example, the *Journal of Psychology and Behavioral Science* published a study in 2015 showing that children who were more optimistic tended to be far more self-efficient and satisfied and subsequently more resilient.[5] Optimism has been shown to enhance resilience by modulating sympathetic tone (i.e. the fight-or-flight aspect of our nervous system), which reduces inflammation, lowers cortisol and ensures stable blood pressure values. Like the Big Five traits, there is a fairly obvious relationship between optimism and resilience promotion. The overlay is such that when we are optimistic *we align our behaviours to a positive future reality* and in doing so create the desired outcome. In other words optimism supports positive actions that culminate in a positive future.

Remarkably, there is a strong molecular component and driving force to the perception and experience of optimism and this is the hormone and neuropeptide oxytocin. Oxytocin is associated with a range of powerful resilience behaviours, including exceptional stress modulation, the promotion of self-belief and even the experience of meaning and purpose.

Oxytocin's broader functional influences and the ways we can engage and enhance this neuropeptide through the foods we eat, the use of nutritional supplements, activities we can perform, environments we need to create for ourselves and, most notably, the behaviours we can take on are explored a bit later in this section.

GENES, PERSONALITY AND FUTURE REALITY

By this point we can appreciate how the genetic make-up of an individual is a considerable factor in intrinsic resilience. Research shows that genetics can impact emotional regulation by at least 20–30 per cent, our temperament in the region of 56 per cent and executive function by as much as 99 per cent.[6] In recent years, geneticists and psychiatrists have been able to identify major gene variants that are associated with greater vulnerability to adverse environments and increased susceptibility to emotional and mental compromise.

But, however insightful, this framework is somewhat rigid and asserts that if you have certain polymorphisms your ability to cope with future challenges and adversity may be compromised, or at the very least limited without medical intervention.

We are more than our coding

Researchers Jay Belsky and Sarah Hartman from the University of California argue against the rigidity of this paradigm, i.e. that an inherited gene variant defines a person's emotional set and future vulnerability[7] and instead reasoned that certain polymorphisms should be conceptualised as "plasticity" rather than "vulnerability" genes.

What this means is that the many gene variants that increase the risk of mental disorders under stressful and challenging conditions can confer significant benefit and be an advantage if we are able to create the right personal conditions for ourselves. In simple terms, if we create an environment that is supportive and caring, practise sound personalised nutrition, exercise regularly, seek enriched learning, have daily sunlight exposure and meditate, the gene risk not only disappears but becomes a significant resilience and performance advantage. In simple terms, our vulnerability may really be our strength.

For example, two of the more recognised "plasticity" genes include 5-HTTLPR, which encodes for a protein that transports serotonin, and, secondly, the dopamine receptor gene, DRD4. These genes were previously recognised by psychiatric geneticists as major vulnerability genes, predisposing carriers of polymorphisms to anxiety, depression, heightened stress reactivity,[8] OCD and attention-deficit hyperactivity disorder (ADHD).[9]

> Many of the genes that increase our risk of mental and emotional issues in response to chronic stress confer benefit under supportive conditions.

However, what Belsky and Hartman were able to show is that these gene variants merely make individuals more sensitive to their surrounding environment and don't necessarily create compromised emotional and mental well-being. In practical terms, what this means is that those children with 5-HTTLPR

> Certain gene variants can make us more sensitive to our environment.

polymorphisms who grow up in a home that has a strong moral compass, who receive love and attention, have responsive parents and live a fairly healthy lifestyle (diet, activity and nature) will adapt, thrive and realise their fullest potential regardless of the challenges that exist in the outside world.

By contrast, those children who experience maltreatment, neglect and antisocial behaviour are more likely to struggle from mental and emotional issues in response to stress and challenges.

> Regardless of one's genetic set or the challenges we face, if we are able to create a home that is encouraging, positive, caring, compassionate and supportive we will be resilient.

The infamous ADHD gene, DRD4, is associated with exceptional behavioural and cognitive outcomes in children when there is robust maternal positivity, when the environment they grow up in is enriched with prosocial behaviours (i.e. care, support, charity, compassion, empathy), early non-familial childcare (building diverse relationships), strong social competence and overall support. On the other hand, children with the same polymorphism who are born on the lower side of birth weight and who experience significant childhood adversity and other ongoing negative stimuli, such as a lack of love, warmth and support, will often struggle with motivation, learning, focus and attention.

> Your weakness may be your strength.

There are no bad genes, only poor environments!

Parents and leaders, let this be our call to action. Our influence on our children and those who fall within our sphere of influence is greater than we could ever imagine. To provide an environment of positivity, encouragement, attentiveness, care, trust, compassion, empathy and support will go a long way in the realisation of their intrinsic potential.

There are at least six known genes (see table on p.47) that make us more sensitive to our environment, both in childhood and later in life.[10] Several years ago, through DNA testing, I discovered that I have polymorphisms in four out of the six genes and am very familiar with the impact of current and historical environments on my resilience and potential.

The primary "plasticity" genes and their role

Gene	Primary behavioural influence	Possible negative effect of the variant in challenging environments	Positive effect under supportive conditions
Brain-derived neurotrophic factor (BDNF)	Promotes memory, retention of information, cognitive ability, creativity, protects against anxiety and depression	Stress-induced emotional vulnerability, reduced cognitive potential, difficulties with learning and reading	Reduced emotional vulnerability to adversity, greater learning potential, enhanced memory (25%) and higher IQ
Oxytocin receptor gene (OXTR)	Reduces the intensity and duration of stress, promotes trust, empathy, self-belief, optimism, courage and sense of calm	Greater stress reactivity, strained relationships, loss of meaning and purpose, increased emotional vulnerability to stress	Exceptional resilience, reduced anxiety and depression, good mental acuity, greater connection to others, enhanced trust and positive self-image
FK506 binding protein 5 (FKBP5)	Has a profound influence on stress perceptions and responses	Increased risk of emotional, behavioural, learning and sleep disorders	Better stress regulation, lower risk of emotional disorders, improved cognitive potential
Monoamine oxidase A (MAOA)	Supports cognitive and emotional integrity by ensuring an optimal balance of dopamine, norepinephrine and serotonin	(Research is ongoing)	(Research is ongoing)
5-HTTLPR	Supports emotional stability (especially under stressful conditions), positive social behaviours and enhanced cognition	Higher vulnerability to adversity, increased risk of anxiety and depression, higher stress reactivity, poorer cognitive functioning in pressure situations later in life	Exceptional resilience, measured emotional responses to stressful events, reduced risk of depression and anxiety
Dopamine receptor D4 (DRD4)	Promotes cognition, augments learning and memory, supports adaptability, regulates emotions and complex behaviours	ADHD, OCD, learning difficulties, impaired memory, impulsivity, thrill-seeking, anger and aggression	Greater adaptability, enhanced cognition and learning, improved problem-solving, stronger memory, lower tendency to anger and higher forgiveness traits

Personal DNA testing

Knowledge is power and, for any resilience journey to be fully supported and enabled, performing a personal DNA analysis will provide you with invaluable information about your genetic make-up. The most important genes to assess include the six vulnerability genes, COMT, as well as prominent genes that reflect immune system behaviours (most notably, interleukin 6 [IL-6]), but there are at least 16 genes that directly influence our response to challenges, predisposition to vulnerability and ultimately our ability to rise above adversity.

Having your DNA tested is very accessible and the service is offered by many biotechnology labs throughout the world. It typically involves a simple buccal (cheek) swab or a blood spot from a finger prick. Once the sample is taken and sent back to the lab, the analysis typically takes 6 to 14 days. The results are summarised in a report that offers basic guidance and direction. Be mindful that it is always advantageous to arrange a consultation with a professional to better interpret the results, and that it is still an emerging science with a way to go.

It is also important to bear in mind that there are a variety of performance panels available that don't assess resilience, but rather general health and wellbeing, sporting potential, medication compatibility and so on. While these can offer valuable insights, it might not be the information you are looking for in a personal actualisation journey.

In 2021 I partnered with DNAlysis in South Africa and dnalife in other countries around the world to develop the first of its kind (and possibly the only) DNA Resilience panel, which places a spotlight on the most influential genes in promoting resilience and unlocking human potential. This deeply insightful information can make future decisions pertaining to optimal lifestyle choices easier, clearer and more effective.

TAKEAWAY MESSAGE

To be resilient in this day and age means that we need to make a personal commitment to develop our self-awareness and engage more with the world around us. This will demand a degree of courage, together with the acknowledgement that there will be some uncomfortable moments along the way as we step out of our comfort zones.

Now is the time to be bold enough to allow our curiosity and imagination to course freely, while at the same time we should aspire towards becoming more structured, self-disciplined and goal-orientated. In this way, our dreams, hopes and passions can be better actualised.

What's more is that we need to progressively build our social confidence and interpersonal warmth. This would all be impossible without considerable effort committed to better regulating our emotions, self-dialogue and the pursuit of serenity.

Finally, we must learn to forgive again. I say again because as young children we neither held onto emotional content nor judged others based on past experiences and disappointments. Every moment was a new opportunity. In this complex and challenging world we find ourselves in as adults, we cannot grow and move forward as over-demanding sceptics, but rather we have to become more selfless, empathetic and forgiving, both of ourselves and others.

SECTION SUMMARY

- Intrinsic personality drives resilience. Traits that include extroversion, openness, agreeableness and conscientiousness are associated with lower vulnerability to adversity.
- Neurotic tendencies detract from resilience.

- Extroversion, openness, agreeableness and conscientiousness are strongly influenced by the neurochemicals dopamine, norepinephrine, oxytocin and serotonin.
- The enzyme COMT has a significant influence on the delicate balance that is needed to ensure neurochemical balance and the optimal expression of self in challenging circumstances.
- To ensure proper expression of COMT it is important to maintain a good supply of B vitamins (B2, B6, B9, B12), either from dietary sources or supplementation. Magnesium glycinate or L-threonate can also be supportive in this regard.
- COMT enzyme levels can be affected by our genetics, behaviours and environment.
- While there are many genetic polymorphisms that are associated with increased vulnerability to adversity, their influence is mitigated, if not altogether reversed, under health-promoting, supportive and nurturing conditions.
- Positive social environments protect against mental and emotional compromise related to significant genetic factors.

LESSON 2

OUR CHILDHOOD FOLLOWS US

Our capacity to be resilient is influenced by several factors outside of us that include the nature of the challenge, at what stage of our life we are exposed to hardship, the duration of the exposure to adversity and the overall intensity of the experience.

Within the context of adversity in children, it most often takes the form of neglect, abuse, a combination of the two, or uncertainty. Sadly, exposure to childhood trauma is more common than we realise or would want to accept. According to researchers from the Department of Health Care Policy and Harvard Medical School, 53.4 per cent of adolescents from high-income countries have experienced childhood adversity in some form.[1]

When looking at low- and middle-income countries, the data is sparse, but all indications suggest that the prevalence of adverse childhood experiences is far higher than this. A southern African study published in 2020 showed that three-quarters of adolescents have suffered four or more adversities.[2]

Moving across the Atlantic to South America, an 18-year observational study of 3,951 Brazilian adolescents showed an 85 per cent prevalence of at least one adverse childhood experience.[3]

The more common events cited by the studies included parental divorce, family violence and abuse (physical, emotional or sexual), neglect (physical or emotional), family economic adversity and parental mental illness. Mental health compromise is one of the greatest challenges the world is currently facing. Parental mental health compromise affects around one in five in high-income countries such as the US,[4] and potentially around one in two in middle-income countries such as Brazil.

■

ADVERSE CHILDHOOD EXPERIENCES TRIGGER MENTAL HEALTH COMPROMISE

Early-life trauma and adversity happen to be two of the most reliable predictors of many common mental health issues, including anxiety, depression, sleep disorders and addiction. In addition, they also play a significant role in contributing to accelerated ageing[5] and premature mortality, especially in women.[6] According to a report by the World Health Organization, drawing data from 21 countries that involved 51,945 participants, 30 per cent of all mental health disorders stem from childhood adversity.[7]

> 30 per cent of all mental health issues stem from childhood adversity.

What is rapidly emerging is an improved awareness and understanding as to how the different early-life adversities, at varied intensities and durations, evoke distinctive degrees of physiological cost, often referred to as allostatic load.

In 2017 a team of researchers from the University of California and Northwestern University identified common elements of childhood adversity that impact child development, which included physical threat, disrupted caregiving and unpredictable environmental conditions.[8] What they aimed to clarify was whether or not there were distinctive biological signatures associated with different types of adversity in adolescents.

> There are distinctive biological signatures associated with different experiences of adversity in childhood.

While it is well established that all childhood adversity has the potential to disrupt both immune and stress hormone responses throughout our lifetime, what the researchers discovered was that different traumas create their unique biological signatures that remain throughout the course of one's lifetime.

Physical abuse and trauma

The 2017 study showed that physical trauma, whether in the form of abuse, surgery or major physical injury, was associated with a disproportionately high activation of the stress axis, namely the hypothalamic-pituitary-adrenal (HPA) axis, together with heightened immune responses that promote chronic systemic inflammation. In other words, following physical abuse, all subsequent stresses (emotional, physical or environmental) are perceived by the body to be greater than they are and the subsequent wear and tear on all biological systems that follows is mostly due to disproportionate and largely dysregulated immune activity.

However, the real health concern, as a consequence of constant over-arousal of the stress axis in response to a life of fear, physical harm and ongoing threat of trauma, is the non-responsiveness of the adrenal glands (the cortisol-producing region of the body) to the adrenocorticotropin hormone (ACTH), a hormone that is central to initiating the stress response. In other words, the body struggles to produce cortisol. Symptoms of low cortisol include depression and anxiety, chronic fatigue, physical weakness, mental confusion, physical pain, rashes, allergies and even an abnormal heart rate.[9]

> If you have experienced a life of adversity and challenges, it may be advantageous to have your doctor evaluate your adrenal function. The Dutch Test offers one of the more comprehensive overviews and is widely available.

Neglect and emotional abuse

In much the same way, physical abuse, trauma and disrupted caregiving has its own biological signature that impacts our resilience in later years. Parental loss, separation, low (or non-existent) parental warmth, neglect and emotional abuse are commonly associated with an inability to regulate cortisol and a reduced ability to normalise the HPA axis throughout your life. In other words, we simply can't shut down our stress axis effectively and the smallest upset can last hours, if not days. This may lead to a variety of ailments, including weight and digestive issues, excessive gastric acid secretion leading to heartburn and reflux, sleep disturbances, repeated injuries and bone abnormalities, changes in the structure and function of the brain, emotional and mental compromise and immune system irregularities.[10]

Uncertainty and feeling unsafe

The same research paper also showed that unpredictable environments, including exposure to violence, accidents, natural disasters (such as the COVID-19 pandemic and the war in Ukraine) and poverty (a reality for millions of people in South Africa and around the world), are associated with hyper-responsiveness of the stress axis. In this heightened state of readiness, everything and anything evokes a stress response, leaving those affected feeling permanently "jumpy" and "on edge", with raised cortisol and inflammation.

The most vulnerable years

Although the negative impact of adverse childhood experiences compromises resilience potential regardless of the age or stage of childhood, the most vulnerable periods appear to be in the first six to 12 months of life, especially in the case of maternal absence, and then again in puberty (particularly as it relates to economic uncertainty).

The following table summarises the independent childhood experiences, but in many instances children experience one or more simultaneously.

The resounding message that can be drawn from this research is that although we have been conditioned to believe that hardship and suffering in childhood create both resilient children and adults, the evidence shows an opposite response. In fact, overwhelming stress and challenges in our formative years often weaken and impair our coping abilities in the future. Rather, future resiliency is best supported by creating an environment that is enriched with diverse activities, healthy foods, one that encourages better sleep, provides all forms of support, promotes a sense of belonging, encourages independence and drives a sense of self-worth and personal value.

Whether you are an adult who came from a challenging background and you are wanting to grow future resiliency, a leader responsible for a team, a teacher overseeing students or a parent trying to create the best possible life for your children, this nurturing model offers a simple template for a bright and successful future for them.

Common stress adaptations in response to childhood adversity

Physical abuse and trauma	Neglect and emotional abuse	Uncertainty and/or constant threat
Disproportional stress responses	Inability to regulate stress responses	Heightened stress reactivity
Chronic inflammation and related disorders	Difficulty calming down following a stressful event	Everything and anything puts one on edge
Adrenal insufficiency disorder (chronic fatigue)		

For those who have experienced neglect, uncertainty or abuse in any context during their formative years, we have the opportunity to start afresh and shape a positive future through the creation and promotion of our own resilient environment. This space could be in your home or at work (preferably both) and should be a place that supports psychological safety and personal growth together with health and overall wellbeing. The following table provides more context.

Supporting family or team resiliency: the top three things I can do

Be a role model	Try to be more emotionally measured and consistent (especially under pressure), show vulnerability and authenticity (i.e. I am a work in progress and have flaws and am actively working on it), be more compassionate and sensitive to others (even when they upset you), and show the courage and conviction pertaining to values and beliefs.
Buffer & protect	Endeavour to create rich social environments that are supportive and promote a sense of belonging. Work on making those around you feel more valued by acknowledging them for the unique contribution to this world and consciously show your appreciation. Finally, encourage independence and accountability.
Support personal growth	Reinforce the importance of high standards, encourage creativity and individuality, and champion enriched and diverse activities. Promote health by placing an emphasis on sleep, nutrition, frequent exercise and periodic relaxation.

SHADES OF GREY – ACUTE CHALLENGE PROMOTES RESILIENCE

Although childhood adversity in the form of neglect, abuse and uncertainty impairs the mental, physical and emotional wellbeing in many of those exposed to it, it is important to realise that stress and challenges are not only important but absolutely necessary in promoting resilience and helping us to reach our potential in life. The distinction is fundamentally the scale, duration of adversity and most importantly the degree of available support. Day-to-day obstacles and trials that don't completely overwhelm our coping mechanisms, when combined with emotional, instrumental and informational support, are immensely facilitative. Examples include the pressure of tests and exams, training and competing in sport, facing daily obstacles, experiencing failure and setbacks, the ongoing demands of education and social skills development.

My grandmother (who was originally from Poland) always held by the notion that "What doesn't kill you, will make you fat'. Unfortunately when it comes to childhood adversity, what "doesn't kill you" may severely impact your wellbeing and resilience later in life. I say this from lived experience.

While they are the exception and not the rule, there are many accounts of children being exposed to hardships and challenges involving one or a combination of physical abuse, neglect and severe unpredictability who are highly resilient. Lucas Radebe, Siya Kolisi and Oprah Winfrey are perfect examples.

How have they overcome such an overwhelming set of odds that life has placed in front of them? The answer is layered, multifactorial and lies with many of the intrinsic factors such as personality and genetics, but it also has to do with what Gin Malhi and his team from the University of Sydney refer to as "tempering" and "reinforcement", concepts that form the basis of the next major learning.

TAKEAWAY MESSAGE

The environment we create for ourselves, our family and our teams ultimately determines resilience. The ideal environment is one where challenges are accompanied by support, care, respect, dignity and ongoing encouragement.

SECTION SUMMARY

- Resilience is largely influenced by the childhood environment we grew up in.
- Sadly, childhood adversities are extremely prevalent both in high- and lower-income countries.
- Mental health compromise later in life is strongly influenced by a history of parental divorce, family violence, abuse, financial uncertainty, parental mental illness and many other adverse childhood experiences.
- The type of adversity we experience as a child has a distinctive emotional and subsequently biological signature later in life.
- While we can't change our past, we have great potential in determining our future. The creation and promotion of healthy, supportive, inclusive and autonomous environments that are enriched with meaning and purpose will go a long way in enhancing our personal resilience.
- Don't fear challenge and adversity. Frequent but short-lived challenges that don't overwhelm coping abilities and that are accompanied by support can be exceptional drivers of resilience.

LESSON 3

NEW CHALLENGES, NEW SKILLS

The word "tempering", when related to resilience, means a process where someone draws off their existing coping skills and further refines or develops them in order to become more resilient in the face of existing and potentially new challenges. Many of these skills and behaviours emerged as powerful and effective survival tools during the more difficult and painful times of our lives. While their value or need at a specific time in our life is not in question, it is important to consider that these traits can arise as highly functional, dysfunctional or somewhere in between.

An all too common dysfunctional form of tempering is when a child who is being subjected to ongoing emotional and psychological abuse builds emotional walls around themselves (albeit temporary) so as to block their pain and hurt and by doing so becomes emotionally distant and disassociated in their personal relationships.

However, if and when they feel emotionally safe (which may never happen), these walls can spontaneously retract, exposing the truest version of self, which is often warm, vulnerable and sensitive. Unfortunately, this state seldom lasts, as the moment the child experiences an emotionally toxic or unsafe environment, whether perceived or real, the armour instantly reappears, often more reinforced and extreme than before. This is often a deeply embedded and subconscious response.

By contrast, there are profoundly positive examples of tempering too. We learn as we get older that the experience of chronic stress, fear and anxiety can be mitigated by, for example, exercise or regular sports participation. In order to cope with abuse, neglect or uncertainty in the home, a child may throw themselves into sports activities, investing a disproportionate amount of time in training, practising and competing. This routine helps them to escape their harsh and sometimes painful realities that exist at home. In time, they may become highly proficient in their chosen sport, opening doors later in life that simply wouldn't have existed otherwise – a story that holds true for many of our sporting heroes.

Beneath the surface lies an additional bouquet of benefits to choosing this path. Through ongoing sport participation, children are able to develop many new and effective resilience skills. These may include the appreciation of the value of support and friendship, the benefit of teamwork, the importance of hard work in promoting success, greater determination, the ability to focus on what matters, greater adaptability, how to better cope with disappointments and setbacks, goal setting and the associated increases in self-confidence and sense of belonging. With every progressive increase in proficiency and competency, i.e. rising up the sporting ladder, the realisation of the value of these skills (i.e. support, teamwork, commitment, determination, etc.) becomes greater and therefore becomes further developed and refined over time.

Seldom do our formative resilience skills fall into positive or negative, functional or dysfunctional, black or white, but rather our reality unfolds as varying degrees of grey. The message one can draw from this is that our future success and personal potency will demand that we work to replace the dysfunctional patterns with more functional ones (not an easy feat) and that our historical coping skills are always in need of an upgrade.

OUR CURRENT SKILLS MAY NOT MAKE THE CUT

A potential issue associated with relying solely on existing skills when facing new challenges (i.e. the process of tempering) is that resilience is in and unto itself heavily reliant on rapid change, perpetual growth, openness and flexibility in thinking as well as significant adaptability. What may happen when we rely too heavily on our pre-existing "survival software" to help us cope is that we are drawing on behaviours and traits that might not be that effective or even relevant in dealing with new and evolving challenges.

Becoming our 2.0 self

To be clear, we should not completely dismiss or diminish the value of the attributes that have helped us navigate a lifetime's worth of stress, challenge and pain. It may be that they are extraordinary in their own right, requiring only subtle enhancements and refinements to suit the existing circumstances.

Our ultimate goal is to grow in the area of self-awareness and gain in personal objectivity – by no means an easy feat. But through our persistent efforts, and with time, we will be able to better identify the necessary skills required for a given challenge and adapt or grow them accordingly.

Upon reflection, the positive skills I took to Beijing were discipline and persistence, but I came to realise that I wasn't using these qualities to their fullest extent. Although I was fairly disciplined with my food choices, exercise and overall health practices, what I needed over and above these basic health behaviours was to be more disciplined with my thoughts and perspectives. This entailed me reminding myself that pressure is a privilege and that no accomplishment that has any meaning or significance whatsoever will be an easy road.

61

Grit, tenacity and persistence are exceptional qualities in themselves and contribute significantly to our success over our lifespan. While they added to my ability to withstand many of the professional, environmental and social stresses in Beijing for months on end, what I needed to learn was to be persistent in other ways, which included building relationships, creating a support structure and constantly reframing my current circumstances.

While the perpetual refinement and development of our personality determines our future success, we need to be aware that tempering (building on existing coping mechanisms) will invariably need to be supported by a commitment to developing new, and sometimes unfamiliar, skills — commonly referred to as reinforcement. For many, this resilience piece is lacking, quite possibly as a result of the difficulty we experience with having to change ourselves and our perspectives.

The COVID-19 pandemic provides the perfect backdrop to explore this framework. Few would argue that the events that began in early 2020 were unlike anything we had experienced before and the socio-political and economic fallout has been nothing short of catastrophic.

According to "Gallup's State of the Global Workforce 2021 Report",[1] a third of workers lost their job (or business) in 2020. At the same time, 80 per cent of those who still held onto employment or their business were completely disengaged and detached. Stress and emotional volatility continue to be major organisational issues, with anger and deep sadness affecting at least one in four team members and chronic stress overwhelming almost half the world's workforce.

Whatever your circumstances, your background or abilities, it would be almost impossible to be resilient under these new socio-economic conditions without drawing on existing coping mechanisms and, more importantly, the acquisition of new skills.

The table on p.64 is a self-reflection and future-orientation tool. I have filled in simple examples based on my perceptions at the time.

Use the blank version of the table on p.65 as an alignment tool for improved resilience awareness and in optimising future direction. An important consideration is that this sheet serves as a call to action in identifying areas that require growth and development in order to support our fullest expression of self, through the challenges that invariably lie ahead.

To bring this concept to life, one must also consider a best practice approach to growing our resilience set. While some answers have been provided especially in the areas of adaptability, openness, agreeableness, extroversion, conscientiousness and optimism, many profound insights and learnings are still to come. My suggestion is to add learnings to those triats that you have identified as a growth opportunity. In practical terms, this may require paging back and forth to this table in order to create the ultimate personal performance solution.

This subjective evaluation can help simplify where it is you need to focus your attention during the more challenging periods of your life. Some of these skills you may have already developed, while others may need to be acquired. This is the dance between tempering and reinforcement that is central to both adolescent and adult resilience.

■

TAKEAWAY MESSAGE

Resilience is fundamentally a set of skills that need to be refined, developed and grown throughout our lives. The key is to identify your primary strengths and leverage off them as much as possible, while at the same time recognising your existing vulnerabilities and consciously working on developing and enhancing them.

Self-reflection and future-orientation sheet

Core resilience traits	Perceived strength (↗) or work in progress (→)	An existing skill/resource	Future Actions
Adaptability and cognitive flexibility	↗ →	In my professional capacity Not as much in my personal capacity	I need to work on this in my personal capacity
Optimism and hope	↗	I am feeling strong	Not at the moment
Openness to new realities and experiences	→	I need constant reminders and strong personal dialogue	Need refinement in this area
Conscientiousness	↗	I am feeling strong	Not at the moment
Agreeableness	→	Room for improvement	I need to work on this in my personal capacity
Motivation and drive	↗	Very focused and driven	Not at the moment
Logic and rational thought	↗	Good but fatigue may undermine it	Need to reduce emotional responses to challenge when fatigued – work to be done
Personal values and beliefs	↗	I am feeling very strong	Keep at it
Emotional regulation	→	Good days and bad days	Need to work a little harder
Goals	↗	I am feeling very strong	May need to develop greater courage to more actively pursue some aspirations
Confidence and self-worth	↗	I am feeling strong	Not at the moment
Coping strategies	↗	I am feeling very strong	Not at the moment
Support system	→	Struggling in this regard	Will need to explore options
Personal health practices	↗	I am feeling very strong	Always opportunity for refinement
Persistence and determination	↗	I am feeling strong	Not at the moment

Core resilience traits	Perceived strength (↗) or work in progress (→)	An existing skill/ resource	Future Actions
Adaptability and cognitive flexibility			
Optimism and hope			
Openness to new realities and experiences			
Conscientiousness			
Agreeableness			
Motivation and drive			
Logic and rational thought			
Personal values and beliefs			
Emotional regulation			
Goals			
Confidence and self-worth			
Coping strategies			
Support system			
Personal health practices			
Persistence and determination			

■

SECTION SUMMARY

- Drawing off existing resilience skills in adversity is typically our default response.
- Oftentimes these skills will need to be further developed and refined in order to promote resilience under varying life–work conditions.
- Often previously developed resilience skills will not offer enough support in an ever-changing world.
- To be resilient we have to embrace the notion that new skills will be required, which will be based on the current challenges and stressors.
- Important resilience skills include adaptability, optimism, openness, conscientiousness, motivation, strong values, emotional regulation, goals, self-confidence, stress regulation, support, health promotion and grit.

LESSON 4

RESILIENCE HAS A DISTINCTIVE SIGNATURE IN THE HUMAN BRAIN

On a purely foundational level, resilience is about the human brain and its ability to successfully adapt both structurally and functionally.

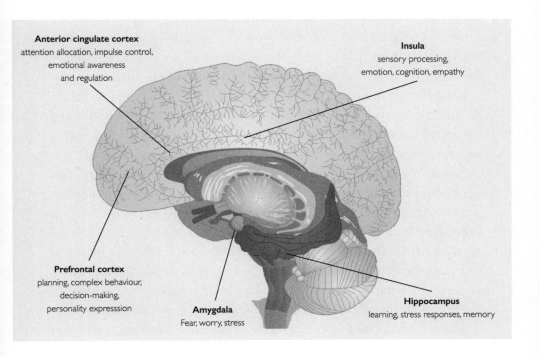

Anterior cingulate cortex
attention allocation, impulse control, emotional awareness and regulation

Insula
sensory processing, emotion, cognition, empathy

Prefrontal cortex
planning, complex behaviour, decision-making, personality expresssion

Amygdala
Fear, worry, stress

Hippocampus
learning, stress responses, memory

This adaptation strongly impacts physiological, cognitive and behavioural responses to acute and chronic stress as well as adversity. Due to the brain being highly plastic and undergoing extensive reorganisation during childhood and adolescence, it is during these periods that resilience can be most effectively developed. However, owing to the brain's dynamic and malleable state, it means not only is it receptive to resilience enhancing, but it also has vulnerability-inducing influences.

LESSENING THE GRIP OF FEAR

Over the last decade there has been an increased interest in neuroimaging studies in order to better understand intra-individual variability in resilience and the development of post-traumatic symptoms or other stress-related disorders. In 2018 researchers from the University of Zurich published a comprehensive review on the neuroimaging correlates of resilience to adversity.[1] The study showed that there are distinct differences in resilient versus vulnerable individuals involving brain volume, connectivity and overall activity in many influential regions, which include the hippocampus, amygdala, insula, anterior cingulate cortex and prefrontal cortex. These regions collectively govern our emotions, ability to learn, stress responses, executive function and sensory processing.

These differences exist in isolated areas but also in larger brain networks, which are regions that show strong functional interdependence. Three of the more influential networks include the default mode network (associated with imagination, self-reflection and cognition), the salience network (drives communication, social behaviour and self-awareness) and the central executive network (promotes problem-solving, maintaining and manipulating information in working memory and goal orientation).

The meta-analysis identified that in more resilient individuals there is greater brain mass in the hippocampus, anterior cingulate cortex and prefrontal cortex. Because greater volume correlates to performance within the brain,[2] it can be deduced that their enhanced resiliency is supported by a greater capacity for attention allocation and focus, decision-making, improved learning ability, enhanced memory, better overall planning, greater impulse control and a stronger moral compass.

Regarding functional connectivity, resilient individuals show reduced connectivity of the fear and emotional centre (the amygdala) to the larger brain networks, specifically the default mode and salience networks. In many respects this significant neural circuit reorganisation loosens the grip of fear and panic in the way we perceive ourselves, how we communicate with others, how we memorise events and how we solve the problems we are confronted with. Without an overwhelming sense of fear and trepidation, we are set free to move forward in life.

Not only does resilience show distinctive patterns that include increased brain mass and a defined change in neural circuitry, there is also a unique trend in brain activity. The research shows that resilient individuals are more effective at consciously and deliberately recruiting the executive regions of the brain, which have the effect of overriding the brain's emotional, stress and fear centres, regardless of circumstances and challenges.

HOW TO CREATE A RESILIENT BRAIN

Many of the structural and functional adaptations that occur within the brain in those who show vulnerability to adversity are associated with prolonged exposure to the stress hormone – cortisol. In 2012 researchers at Yale University identified that at least seven regions of the brain atrophy in response to chronic stress and cortisol exposure.[3] At the same time, a study at the University of California showed that prolonged cortisol exposure causes stem cells to malfunction, resulting in altered composition and connectivity within the brain.[4]

Whether raised cortisol is a result of chronic stress and adversity, the scale and magnitude of the immediate challenge, existing genetic vulnerabilities (specifically FKBP5 and Corticotropin-releasing hormone receptor 1 [CRHR1]), lousy timing of life's challenges (i.e. in childhood and adolescence) or a combination of any of these factors, it can be successfully managed and its negative effects on resilience can be completely mitigated.

In order to combat chronically raised cortisol and its negative effects on the brain and consequently, resilience, two simple interventions offer immeasurable benefits and protection. These include increasing your intake of omega-3 fatty acids (through food choices or preferably supplementation) and the ancient practice of meditation.

Omega-3 fatty acids

Marine-derived omega-3 fatty acids containing eicosapentaenoic acid (EPA) and docosahexaenoic acid (DHA) are believed to be the single most important nutrient complex in the human diet, contributing significantly to mental, emotional and physical performance. The best sources of omega-3 fatty acids include herring, mackerel, sardines, anchovies, wild salmon, walnuts and flax and chia seeds. Sadly, with our modern diet preferences, together with food processing, around 80 per cent of the world's population may not be consuming enough of this oil to meet basic biological needs.[5]

Lowers stress perception

Research into omega-3 fatty acids and stress dates back decades. In 2003 French and Swiss researchers discovered that a robust daily dose of omega-3 fatty acids is able to significantly diminish stress responses (i.e. raised cortisol, adrenaline, etc.).[6] Remarkably, this shift can take place in a very short time span (under three weeks).

Protects the brain

In 2016 the *International Journal of Neuropsychopharmacology* published a study on the relationship between stress hormones, omega-3 fatty acids (specifically DHA) and brain composition. In the animal study it showed that when cells from the brain's executive region (frontal cortex) are exposed to cortisol for a period exceeding 48 hours they become structurally compromised and die.[7]

Cells from the frontal cortex are particularly sensitive to the influence of cortisol due to a high density of glucocorticoid receptors (proteins which mediate its effects). Incredibly, when pre-treated with omega-3 fatty acids, the neurons were completely immune to the damaging effects of cortisol. The message that can be drawn from this research, and the many other studies like it, is that higher dietary intakes of omega-3 fatty acids, over protracted periods of time, has the potential to support optimal brain structure and function regardless of the challenges we may be confronted with at the time.

Augments cognitive potential

Yet another benefit attributed to optimal intakes of omega-3 fatty acids is the increased expression of BDNF. BDNF is a protein produced inside nerve cells that promotes the structural integrity and functionality of the brain through new brain cell formation, maturation and retention, as well as by building connections between the cells. Through a variety of mechanisms, BDNF is the basis for brain cell integrity and functionality, as well as cognitive and possibly even behavioural potential.

In 2014 a team of German researchers published a human study showing that ongoing supplementation with omega-3 fatty acids results in significant cognitive improvements, largely through elevations in BDNF.[8] The study involved 65 healthy subjects who were given either 2.2 grams of fish oil, or a placebo, for a period of 26 weeks. A large range of tests were performed before and after the intervention, including cognitive performance assessments and neuroimaging. The findings showed that those subjects who supplemented with omega-3 fatty acids

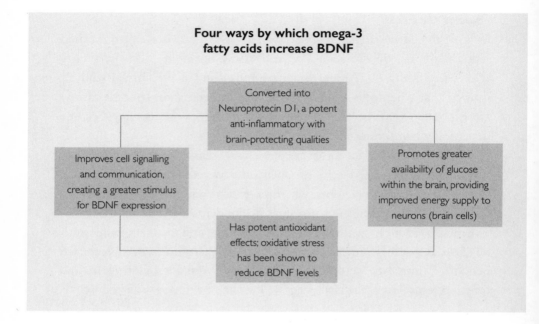

Four ways by which omega-3 fatty acids increase BDNF

Converted into Neuroprotecin D1, a potent anti-inflammatory with brain-protecting qualities

Improves cell signalling and communication, creating a greater stimulus for BDNF expression

Promotes greater availability of glucose within the brain, providing improved energy supply to neurons (brain cells)

Has potent antioxidant effects; oxidative stress has been shown to reduce BDNF levels

experienced an increase in brain mass in several key regions and showed dramatically enhanced cognition.

Animal studies show that 12 days of an omega-3-fatty-acid-enriched diet was able to raise BDNF by 125 per cent in the absence of exercise and by 144 per cent when combined with regular activity.[9]

How much should you take for general health and improved resilience?

The standard dietary recommendations for omega-3 fatty acids is 250–500 mg per day for health promotion and protection.[10] For individuals who have no underlying medical conditions, the National Institutes of Health recommends 1.1 grams per day for adult women, 1.6 grams per day for adult men and 500–900 mg for children aged six months to nine years. From the age of nine to 18, doses are fairly close to the adult range.[11]

Foods high in omega-3 fatty acids

Food	Quantity	Omega-3 fatty acids
Salmon	100g	2.5g
Mackerel	100g	2.78g
Herring	100g	2.67g
Anchovies	100g	2.2g
White fish	100g	1.9g
Tuna (canned)	100g	0.9g
Sea bass	100g	0.9g
Flax seeds	100g	23g*
Chia seeds	100g	17.8g*
Walnuts	100g	9g*

Source: https://www.myfooddata.com/articles/high-omega-3-foods.php

* It is important to consider that while these foods are extremely high in omega-3 fatty acids, they may not be biologically available and therefore not preferable. Plant sources of omega-3 fatty acids contain alpha-linolenic acid (ALA) as opposed to the marine sources that contain EPA and DHA. At least seven intervention studies show that ALA is not converted into DHA. As a vegetarian or vegan, supplementation with marine algae may be the best option.[12] Moreover, there are significant genetic variations in the metabolism of omega-3 fatty acids, meaning that some individuals will struggle to acquire enough through traditional dietary means and need to supplement in order to optimise health and personal resilience. A genetic test (e.g. DNA health test offered by reputable biotechnology labs) focusing on general health will clarify vulnerabilities in this area.

Depression and anxiety

Due to the impact of adversity and chronic stress on the brain inflammatory pathways, levels of serotonin, BDNF, dopamine, GABA (gamma amino-butyric acid) and other neurochemicals, it should come as no surprise that a robust negative correlation exists in the domain of mental health.

What is fascinating to scientists is the relationship between levels of DHA in the executive regions and the experience of major depression. It has been shown that those suffering from major depression typically show 22 per cent lower levels of DHA within these regions of the brain, compared to those in normal control groups.

A 2015 randomised placebo-controlled trial involving 23 young participants who were suffering with depression were given either 1.4 grams of
omega-3 fatty acids or an equal-sized capsule of corn oil.[13] After 21 days,
the researchers re-evaluated both groups and to their astonishment there
was a significant difference between the groups, in that 67 per cent of
those taking the fish oil no longer fitted the criteria for depression.

In another study, a group of 68 medical students were given 2.5 grams
of omega-3 fatty acids or a placebo and carefully evaluated (including
blood analysis), both under stressful conditions and in periods of relative
calm.[14] What the researchers found was that compared to controls, those
given omega-3 fatty acids showed a 20 per cent reduction in anxiety and
significantly reduced inflammation.

Supplementation

For many of us, the regular consumption of contamination-free cold-water
fish may neither be practical nor preferable (i.e. for those with fish allergies,
vegetarians, from an affordability perspective or other factors such as wishing
to avoid methylmercury contamination). In this instance, supplementation
is a wise and easy solution. There are countless products on the market
advertising and promoting their efficacy. When selecting a supplement, as
a rule of thumb, choose products that are derived from sardines, mackerel,
herring and anchovies, as these are non-predatory, non-bottom-feeding fish
and are generally lower in environmental contaminates (methylmercury,
polychlorinated biphenyls, dioxins and organochlorines). If you are vegan,
microalgae (phytoplankton)is the best option.

Ideally, the product you choose should be sustainably sourced and
certified by third-party labs such as the National Sanitation Foundation
(NSF) to ensure potency, purity and freshness.

*A word of caution:

If you are taking anticoagulants (medication used to reduce blood clotting)
avoid taking high doses of omega-3 supplements as it may lead to bleeding

Resilience influence of omega-3 fatty acids and ideal dosing

Action	Men	Women	Children (<9)	Adolescents (>9)
Restore health	250–500 mg/day	250–500 mg/day	250–500 mg/day	250–500 mg/day
Improve health	1.6 grams/day	1.1 grams/day	500–900 mg	1–1.6 grams
Manage depression	1.6 grams/day	1.4 grams/day	No established dose	No established dose
Manage anxiety	2.5 grams/day	2.5 grams/day	No established dose	No established dose
Lower inflammation	2.5 grams/day	2.5 grams/day	No established dose	No established dose
Enhance brain structure and improve cognition	2.2 grams/day	2.2 grams/day	No established dose	No established dose
Alter stress responses	1.6–2.5 grams/day	1.5–2.5 grams/day	No established dose	No established dose

issues. Other issues that can arise from high doses of supplemental omega-3 fatty acids include acid reflux, diarrhoea and low blood pressure. Should you experience any of these side effects, speak to your healthcare practitioner for guidance.

Meditation

In recent years there have been a plethora of studies investigating alterations in brain structure (morphology) corresponding to meditation practice in adults.[15] For example, a meta-analysis of 21 neuroimaging studies of experienced meditation practitioners found that at least eight regions of the brain showed increased grey matter volume and concentration, as well as cortical thickness as a consequence of meditation practice. The regions that showed enlargement are those that influence awareness, memory, inter-hemispheric communication and emotional regulation – all positive resilience promotors.

In a small Italian study published in the journal *Brain Behaviour*, 45 students were randomly assigned to a meditation or a control group.[16] The meditation group had no prior experience and was subjected to four open-monitoring practice sessions a week that lasted a duration of 45–50 minutes each for a period of a month. Open-monitoring meditation emphasises developing an open and accepting attitude and learning to let go of mental content, neither resisting nor elaborating on anything that surfaces in your awareness. For most of us, this requires considerable practice to be able to achieve this state, as rumination is all too common.

The intention of the study was to fill a gap in the research with a longitudinal randomised controlled design by assessing the effect of a four-week, open-monitoring meditation training on grey matter density and intrinsic brain activity.

The researchers found that within the meditation group and within a period of under a month (involving less than 20 hours of active meditation participation), subjects displayed an improvement in self-perceived general wellbeing and showed a significant change in brain structure and intrinsic activity in the inferior fronto-insular regions (those areas associated with executive control) when compared to the control group. What the research team also uncovered was an active reorganisation and enhancement of the central executive network, the network commonly recruited by tasks requiring controlled information processing, flexibility and working memory.

Least amount of effort for greatest return

Although many of studies that have focused on the structural and functional benefits of meditation were performed over several months (sometimes years) and typically involved longer sessions lasting 45–60 minutes, the reality is that the benefits of meditation can be realised with far less practice.

A 2017 study published in *Frontiers in Systems Neuroscience* had 25 university students who had no prior experience in meditation perform ten 30-minute mindfulness meditation sessions over a period of two weeks.[17] All the participants were exposed to extensive neuroimaging prior to and following the intervention. It was discovered that within the two weeks, 60 new functional connections appeared in key brain circuits responsible for supporting attention, cognitive and emotional processing, awareness and sensory integration and reward processing. In other words, five hours of meditation over two weeks was able to dramatically improve brain structure and function. Outside of regular exercise, there is no other activity, medication, supplement, food or behaviour that offers this level of neurological benefit.

Selecting a meditation practice

The first step in a personal meditation journey is to choose the type or style of meditation that you feel you will able to connect to, is easy and, most importantly, that you will enjoy. Some forms of meditation create a target for attention, some create a mantra, others a dialogue or a focus on letting go. Bear in mind that you needn't be locked into any particular method as you can interchange between the various practices at any stage. Below is a short synopsis of the different types of meditation and their highly nuanced benefits.

Focused-based practices

Focused-based meditation places an emphasis on highly focused attention, which typically involves minimal distraction while observing the breath. The nature of the practice is to highlight concentration and introspection.

According to an article published in *Trends in Cognitive Sciences*, focused attention meditation can enhance attention, disengage from distraction and shift attention back to its intended target, as well as improve skills in the area of cognitive reappraisal.[18] This meditation practice is associated with increased dopamine and improved signalling.

Personal application:
✓ Increase and enhance focus, concentration and attention
✓ Reduce vulnerability to distraction in disruptive environments

Loving kindness

This can be a particularly valuable form of meditation for those who are susceptible to negative self-dialogues or who have experienced adverse events and are still entangled in challenges from an emotional and psychological standpoint. The goal of loving kindness is to deepen feelings of sympathetic joy for all living beings (including yourself) as well as promote altruistic behaviours.

This meditative practice can be effective in developing empathy for others, promoting pro-social behaviour and in elevating oxytocin.[19] Moreover, research shows that loving kindness (or any compassion-based meditation) impacts regions of the brain involved in emotional intelligence, sensory information, language and mathematical capabilities.[20]

Personal application:
✓ Strengthen communication skills, ability to connect to others more effectively
✓ Enhance mathematical capabilities

Mindfulness or open monitoring

This form of meditation emphasises developing an open and accepting attitude and learning to let go of mental content, neither resisting nor elaborating on anything that surfaces in your awareness. It also requires the regulation of attention in order to maintain focus on the immediate experience such as thoughts, emotions, body posture and physical sensations, as well as the ability to approach these experiences with a level of openness and acceptance.

Open-monitoring meditation practices increase activity in the brain and enhance the regions that are responsible for movement potential, the processing of emotional content as well as memory and learning.

Personal application:
✓ Improve emotional regulation
✓ Enhance memory and learning
✓ Support movement or physical skill development

Where to start?
There are many ways to engage in meditation practice and some of these include:

- Guided instruction by a trained professional, which is always the best option when first starting out.
- The use of apps such as Calm, Headspace and Breathe.
- Participation in meditation courses or programmes such as mindfulness-based stress reduction.
- Watching tutorials on YouTube.
- Joining a yoga or meditation class.

With all the options available, the decision as to which direction you are going to take in your meditation practice will ultimately depend on the level of enjoyment, time availability and budget.

How often, how long?
Meditation can be transformative with as little as two sessions a week, but ideally it should become a daily practice. To date there is no prescription for optimal meditation duration, but research shows that as little as 12 minutes a day can positively alter genetic behaviours in favour of reduced inflammation.[21] Another study on meditation showed that 13 minutes a day for eight weeks improved mood state, attention, working memory, recognition memory as well as decreased anxiety.[22] This said, most of the research supporting all

the positive improvements involve sessions ranging from 30 to 45 minutes. Knowing this, you have to do what feels right for you. On the days you are pressed for time, find a 12–13 minute gap and on the days that you do have the time, carve out the space and opt for longer sessions.

TAKEAWAY MESSAGE

The health of our brain determines our resilience potential. Supporting the brain structure and function through the intake of omega-3 fatty acids, regular meditation and effective stress management is important, especially during the more challenging periods of our lives.

SECTION SUMMARY

- Resilient individuals:
  - have greater brain mass and improved performance in the regions of the brain that support attention and focus, decision-making, learning, memory, planning, impulse control and even ethics and values.
  - show reduced connectivity between the stress centres and the major brain networks that govern imagination, cognition, social behaviour and self-awareness (the default mode and salient networks).
  - recruit the executive regions of the brain more effectively and also show executive/cognitive control over emotion.
- Chronic stress and raised cortisol results in brain atrophy, impaired connectivity and stem cell malfunction that compromises resilience and increases vulnerability to adversity.

- To promote resilience, it is important to support and reinforce structural and functional integrity within the brain. This can be achieved by daily consumption of marine-derived omega-3 fatty acids and through regular meditation practice.
- Marine-derived omega-3 fatty acids support resilience by reducing stress responses and emotional reactivity, protecting the brain from cortisol-related damage and by increasing BDNF expression.
- Daily intake of omega-3 fatty acids can reduce the perception of stress in less than three weeks.
- 1.4–2.5 grams of omega-3 fatty acids may reduce depression and anxiety.
- 20 hours a month of meditation dramatically enhances brain structure.
- Five hours of meditation within a period of two weeks increases neuroplasticity and supports improved attention and awareness, as well as cognitive and emotional processing.
- To experience the resilience benefits of meditation, it is important to create a daily habit that is relatively easy, enjoyable and relatable.
- As little as 12–13 minutes a day of meditation has been shown to enhance genetic behaviours, reduce immune activity and lower inflammation, improve memory, attention and focus as well as decrease anxiety.

LESSON 5

INTELLECT DRIVES RESILIENCE

Positive regulation of our emotional state is fundamental to resilience and to successful adaptation to ever-changing and ever-demanding realities. Learning to acknowledge, regulate and control our emotional set (that includes both experience and response) is very much a self-directed process where the ultimate goal is to positively influence the intensity, duration and type of emotion being experienced. In simple terms, we need to learn to get a grip on our emotions in order to be more successful.

This should not be confused with emotional repression (something I became a master of in my younger years), where we or social factors (parents, teachers, friends, bosses, colleagues) around us allow little wiggle room to experience and express how we feel. Not validating our emotional experiences can be painful and extremely stressful, leading to an internal storm of negative emotions, which will eventually lead to adverse psychological, physical or social outcomes. Instead, emotional regulation relies on greater self-awareness and reflection, acknowledgement of experiences, a constructive approach to self-restraint and the ability to broaden our focus aperture. In other words, we need to develop and refine the habit of thinking with a clear head.

While there are numerous factors that govern our emotional state in response to adversity, which include our current state of health (when we feel unwell we tend to be more emotional and reactive), neurochemistry, genetic make-up, environment and past experiences, it is important to consider that, at its core, emotional responses (whether suppressed, regulated or heightened) to events and challenges are hugely influenced by perception.

How we perceive the world around us tends to create that very reality. This is because our biological, neurochemical and behavioural responses follow our perspective at that specific point in time.

Our thoughts become our words, our words become our actions and our actions shape our reality.

For most, the ability to consciously and more positively alter our perception of events does typically develop with age and life experience. As we get older, we come to realise that challenge and adversity (as opposed to trauma or tragedy) is often momentary or may in fact have a silver lining somewhere in the distant future. This constantly evolving skill (the ability to have a positive perspective in challenging situations) has the potential to promote significant emotional regulation and with it tremendous resilience at any stage of life. That said, the younger we develop this resilience skill, the greater the positive influence during the course of our lives and our ability to handle adversity as adults.

■

REPRESSION, RUMINATION AND AVOIDANCE MAKE US MORE VULNERABLE

Reframing, also known as cognitive reappraisal, is the ability to evaluate our thoughts and replace negative ones with positive ones. It requires a conscious reassessment or reinterpretation of life's setbacks and challenges to consistently find a positive perspective. Research shows that compared to all other common emotional regulation strategies, including rumination, avoidance, suppression and problem-solving, reappraisal is associated with the lowest risk of mental health compromise in response to adversity.[1]

Yet, for some reason our default responses to stress tends to be rumination, avoidance and emotional inhibition. Take a moment to reflect on how many times you have experienced a distributive injustice (i.e. not felt acknowledged, valued or rewarded for your efforts), either in the workplace or in a social setting, and have replayed the event/s over and over again to such an extent that it has impacted your sleep and wellbeing for days on end. Or alternatively, how often has someone or something upset you and your default reaction is to avoid the person or situation in an attempt to suppress the overwhelming feelings of anger and resentment? I can't count the number of times this has been my default strategy and, in all instances, it has been to my detriment.

Unfortunately, these all-too-common defences corrode our own emotional and mental wellbeing and in no way support adaptability and future success. There are many learnt strategies that can be used (consciously or subconsciously) in reframing events and some of these valuable examples are expanded on below.

Psychological distancing

This involves focusing on ways to separate yourself from sources of stress by increasing the distance between yourself and an upsetting cue. For example, an aspiring tennis player may receive negative feedback on their technique or tactics used during a match from their coach and team. In many instances this feedback follows a loss or setback and is certainly not what a player wants to hear at that moment. However, if they train themselves to create a certain degree of emotional distance from the feedback, they are then able to realise that it is not personal criticism but a strategy and vehicle for ongoing growth improvement. By realising that the failure on the day was not a personal shortcoming, but rather a step towards refinement and mastery of learnt skills and trained abilities, the player is able to fully benefit from the experience.

Lewis Hamilton is widely regarded as the greatest Formula 1 driver in the history of the sport. He has won 103 races and the World Driver Championship on seven occasions. Hamilton is a master not only on the track but in the area of psychological distancing too. Where most other drivers see their failures and shortcomings as major inadequacies or deficiencies in personal competency, Hamilton sees his failures as enablers of greater personal accomplishments: "I have failed more times than I can remember. But the lessons that I've learnt through those failures have ultimately ended up with me having success. It's character building. It's where I hone in on my strengths or where I build strength," he says.

It is not to say that Hamilton doesn't have those moments where he questions his abilities and journey – like the rest of us he does. But through many years of practice (he started racing when he was eight years old) and repetition in psychological distancing, he is able to bounce back and move forward.

According to Hamilton: "Failure, in my opinion, failure is 100 per cent necessary for greatness. To achieve greatness, to have that success, you've got to fail as many times as possible. So don't shy away from it. And don't take it as a negative. Every single successful person who's achieved great things, whether it's climbing Mount Everest, whether it's getting to a top of a company, whether it's being the best athlete possible, they've all failed more times than they'll be able to remember. But through those lessons that they've learnt through those failures, that's how they've become great." As powerful as this cognitive strategy is, other more behaviourally and less functionally oriented forms of reframing do exist. Challenging reality and changing circumstances are examples.

Children as young as four years of age can successfully engage in psychological distancing and doing so has been shown to improve their performance on cognitively demanding or frustrating tasks.[2]

Challenging reality

This prominent strategy is used in reframing. When challenging reality, people tend to promote and support the belief that the adverse experience is not entirely real. For example, a marriage that has broken down. Not wanting to confront the issue, which would require repairing or dissolving the relationship, both parties pretend that everything is okay and they "carry on as usual'. Over time they become increasingly estranged and the relationship becomes more dysfunctional. While challenging reality will improve emotional regulation for the duration of the breakdown, it is more of a behaviourally focused strategy as opposed to a cognitively mediated one. In simple terms, although temporarily effective on an emotional level, it is certainly not the best reframing strategy in the long run, from a resilience and self-actualisation perspective.

Changing circumstances

This method of reframing means we reinterpret the details of events to make them appear less negative. For example, during the COVID-19 lockdowns many individuals, teams and families chose to focus on the benefits of being at home (i.e. more family time, no daily commute, home exercise) as opposed to fixating on the more prominent issues like amplified financial pressures, vastly reduced professional growth opportunities and the total collapse of social networks, both personally and professionally. While it can be a powerful resilience skill, one must be very careful not to completely dismiss or diminish the existing challenges in the process, as this may lead to emotional repression and a lack of validation of emotional experiences.

I have personally used both challenging reality and changing circum-stances in order to overcome negative thoughts and replace them with positive perspectives. While these strategies did support me at the time, they are less functional approaches (especially in the case of challenging reality) and cannot be compared to many of the other positive reframing strategies outlined elsewhere in this book.

It's not what we say but how we say it

Research shows that the degree to which someone has adopted cognitive reappraisal can be measured through psycholinguistics. Our choice of words reflects our capacity to reframe an adverse event and the state of our emotional and mental state at the time of the experience.

The use of words that refer to ourselves (I, me, my) and words that refer to the present moment (e.g. angry, frustrated, irritated) indicate that a person is entirely focused on the "here and now", whereas less use of these word classes indicates a more distanced and logical perspective.

According to a study done by Harvard researchers in 2017,[3] when we carefully select our words in response to a stressful event by describing the event as if we were far away (physical distancing), without using the word "I" (social distancing) or without using verbs in the present tense (mental and emotional distancing), it spontaneously reduces the negative effects of the event.

Psycholinguistics also influences resilience potential as we are able to remove ourselves (I, me, my) from external events and adversity, and the challenges become less about our failures and shortcoming and more directed towards finding future solutions.

At the same time, by not using present tense verbs that reflect a current (and often future) reality, we consciously or subconsciously create a psychological state of optimism and hope by placing the struggle in the past.

A failed pitch to a potential client is a perfect opportunity to change the narrative in terms of our response to a disappointing performance. You go into the presentation knowing you have an incredible offering that will do well to support the business you're pitching to; however, during the meeting you struggle to communicate your vision effectively and simply. Perhaps you rambled too much, didn't answer the potential client's questions with confidence or were too nervous to be articulate. Following the failed pitch, you feel upset with yourself for not having delivered successfully. A non-resilient and destructive self-dialogue would be: "I messed this up. I rambled too much, I was so stressed, I didn't listen ... I always make these mistakes. I'm really terrible at sales."

But a resilient and constructive approach would be: "This wasn't the best pitch. The three things that can be improved going forward are: listening skills, stress management and greater simplicity in the messaging. Sales may not be a strength just yet, but it's only a matter of time."

GETTING THE BALL ROLLING

Positive reappraisal can be successfully learnt and applied at any age or stage of life. Whether you choose to psychologically distance, challenge circumstances or use directed word usage, it is the most important resilience skill that, at its centre, focuses on developing self-awareness and self-mastery.

To help you reappraise adverse situations, ask yourself the following questions:

1. What can I learn/gain from this challenge/obstacle?
2. Could there be positive outcomes from this situation in the future?
3. How has this challenge refined, enhanced or strengthened me?
4. What could the greater meaning be beneath the challenge?
5. Am I being proactive or reactive in this situation?
6. Am I open to a new reality?
7. What could I do better tomorrow to help me move forward?

A central theme that emerges from the research into resilience in both children and adults is that the more we are able to draw off high-level cognitive function, i.e. attention, problem-solving, learning and working memory, the greater the potential for adaptability and enhanced realisation of intrinsic potential.

CREATING THE RIGHT NEUROCHEMISTRY TO REFRAME

Developing and refining the skill of reframing is slightly more complex than practice and ongoing commitment to the habit. Rather, a very specific neurochemical equilibrium must be present, especially in the executive regions of the brain (prefrontal cortex). This balance relies on optimal levels of catecholamines, neurochemicals and hormones that are typically associated with stress responses. These include dopamine, norepinephrine and epinephrine. Collectively they are involved in many facets of our personality that encompass drive, motivation, persistence, behaviour and memory consolidation. COMT, an enzyme previously discussed within the framework of resilient personality traits like extroversion, openness, consciousness and agreeableness, is the primary enzyme in the prefrontal cortex that metabolises catecholamines. Any alteration in COMT activity (which has strong genetic influences) will affect dopamine, norepinephrine and epinephrine levels, impacting cognitive and emotional states as well as stress responses.[4] Gene inheritance strongly determines whether or not we have low, medium or high enzymatic activity, which in turn impacts cognitive reappraisal potential. As previously mentioned, variances in dopamine metabolism, depending on your genetic set, can be as much as 300–400 per cent.[5]

In 2018 a team of researchers from Stanford, Columbia and Harvard universities, headed up by psychologist Alia Crum, looked at a specific COMT variation and whether or not it had the potential to modify emotional and cognitive responses to stress.[6] What the research team found was that those individuals who had the lower activity gene variant, and therefore higher dopamine levels within the brain, were able to successfully reframe stress, challenges and adversity. In addition, what flowed from the raised catecholamines was dramatically enhanced cognitive functioning and a happiness bias in response to challenges.

By contrast, for those individuals who were born with the high activity gene variant and consequently lower dopamine levels within the brain, the cognitive reappraisal of stressful events proved extremely difficult and their overall perception of stress and negative events was debilitating.

I have experienced this contrast many times when engaging with businesses, sports teams or even students. While there are countless individuals that have been able to successfully recalibrate their perspective through adversity using cognitive reappraisal, there have been others (approximately 40 per cent) who, no matter how clear and defined the reframing narrative is and how often it is reiterated, simply can't adapt their mindset in their difficult and challenging moments.

Paradoxically, resilience is not entirely supported by enzyme activity and raised dopamine levels either. Studies show that those individuals who have intrinsically higher dopamine (due to reduced COMT activity), and who don't reframe stressful and challenging events, are more likely to experience impaired cognition and tremendous emotional and physical reactivity, which includes increased anxiety, neuroses, depression and raised cortisol.[7]

The fact that dopamine (or any of the catecholamines for that matter) on its own doesn't translate into improved resilience is testament to the power of our choice over our behaviour in shaping current and future realities. By deliberately creating a mindset that sees challenges as opportunities for growth and ultimate success, genetically driven elevations in catecholamines can be channelled in such a way that they create a resilience superpower.

Stanford's Alia Crum found that in those with inherently higher dopamine levels, the impact of cognitive reframing is so profound that when compared to those who didn't reframe, cognitive performance under stressful conditions was 300 per cent greater, with the risk of emotional vulnerability all but disappearing. This is one of the reasons genetic testing can be very helpful in every resilience journey, as it can create greater personal awareness pertaining to those behaviours or activities that offer the greatest value or benefit to our mental, emotional and physical wellbeing.

If you have already performed a genetic test and have inherited the low dopamine variant or if you haven't explored your genetic make-up but really struggle with cognitive reappraisal and finding positive perspectives when exposed to adverse experiences, it may be advantageous to incorporate practices that reduce COMT enzyme expression and/or activity.

There are two simple ways to achieve this, which support your health at the same time:

■ Get moving

Aerobic-orientated exercise (around three sessions for 45–50 minutes per week) has been shown to significantly reduce the activity and levels of COMT.[8] At the same time, aerobic exercise increases dopamine expression and improves its effects within the brain. Whether you choose to walk, run, swim, cycle, play tennis or soccer, row or hike, the key is to just do it – and regularly.

■ Supplement with Bacopa monnieri

Bacopa monnieri – also known as Water hyssop or Brahmi – has been used in traditional Ayurvedic medicine for thousands of years. Bacopa monnieri has exceptionally strong adaptogenic properties, i.e. it can increase the body's ability to resist the damaging effects of stress and promote or restore normal physiological functioning. It is typically prescribed for anxiety, depression, learning disorders, memory decline, inflammation, pain, fevers, blood disorders and even heavy-metal poisoning.

A 2016 study by Indian researchers showed that Bacopa monnieri is a potent inhibitor of COMT[9] and can therefore be especially beneficial for those genetically predisposed to over-expression.

Bacopa monnieri: how to take it and what to look out for

Nutrient	Dose	Indications	Reasons not to take	Goes well with
Bacopa monnieri	300 mg/day	An inability to reframe stress and adversity Genetic polymorphisms in COMT (over-expression)	Genetic polymorphisms in COMT (under-expression), if you suffer from thyroid issues; if you are taking medication for Alzheimer's disease or dementia, or if you have liver or intestinal enzyme insufficiencies, most notability cytochrome P450 3A4 (CYP3A4)	Food that contains fats

The standard dose for Bacopa monnieri is 300 mg per day.[10] Bacopa monnieri is fat soluble and therefore requires a lipid transporter to be absorbed effectively. It should be taken with a meal containing a high proportion of fats (e.g. nuts, olive oil, seeds, eggs). Bacopa is well tolerated by most people, with few known side effects apart from stomach upset, which can be reduced by consuming it with food.

■

SECTION SUMMARY

- Emotional regulation and control are fundamental to resilience.
- Our emotional state is governed by several factors, which include our current state of health, neurochemistry, genetics, environment and past experiences.
- The greatest influence on our emotional state and reactivity to events is the way we perceive the world around us.
- Creating a positive perception of negative events (cognitive reappraisal) is a learnt skill.

- Cognitive reappraisal (reframing) is the ability to evaluate one's thoughts and replace negative ones with positive ones.
- Cognitive reappraisal surpasses rumination, suppression and even problem-solving in protecting us against mental health compromise.
- Psychological distancing involves the conscious separation of oneself from a stressor.
- Challenging reality is an emotional coping mechanism where we create a belief that an adverse experience doesn't really exist and, while it is effective, it may not be conducive to supporting personal growth and long-term resilience.
- Changing circumstances is a method of reframing where one reinterprets the details of a stressful event and makes it appear less negative.
- Our choice of words (psycholinguistics) reflects our level of resilience.
- The use of words that refer to oneself (I, me and my), together with words that refer to the present moment, suggest a greater level of emotional entanglement in current events and consequently a higher degree of vulnerability.
- Our choice of words not only distances us from existing challenges but also makes us more solution-orientated and optimistic.
- In order to reframe successfully we need to ensure optimal levels and function of catecholamines (dopamine, epinephrine and norepinephrine).
- The biggest influence over catecholamine levels is the enzyme COMT.
- Raised levels of dopamine supports cognitive reappraisal, enhanced cognitive functioning and even happiness bias under challenging circumstances.
- The combination of raised dopamine and cognitive reappraisal can improve cognitive performance by 300 per cent.
- If you struggle to reframe adverse events, it may be advantageous to reduce COMT enzyme activity through regular engagement in aerobic activity (45–60 minutes, three times a week) and/or by supplementing with Bacopa monnieri.

LESSON 6

THE POWER OF SUPPORT
AND CONNECTION

The human stress response is immeasurably powerful. The mere perception of a threat or challenge is enough to engage numerous regions of the brain (e.g. amygdala, hypothalamus and pituitary) and cause a five-fold surge of norepinephrine and epinephrine in our bodies. This takes place before our visual system has even had time to register the events happening around us. At the same time, there is a surge of hormones and proteins (neuropeptides) that ultimately trigger an enormous shift in neurological, metabolic and immune behaviours.

The stress axis is the body's survival software that has effectively protected us against unimaginable threats for thousands of years. It is a "software program" where four major systems become drastically enhanced (immune, cardiovascular, hormonal and nervous) in real time, giving us a range of abilities that can be likened to superpowers. In an acutely stressed state, physical strength and explosiveness, endurance, mental acuity, focus and attention, pain resistance and abundant energy combine with heightened senses, providing a vehicle for incredible accomplishment. But as the saying goes – there are no free lunches.

This large-scale biological reorganisation is extremely taxing and can't be sustained for long periods or with great frequency without an overwhelming cost to our emotional, mental and physical wellbeing. In fact, chronic or repeated activation of the stress axis will invariably lead to dysfunction, which may include overactivity, blunted responses, an inability to regulate responses and failure to shut down. It is fair to say that a significant percentage of the world's mental and physical health challenges stems from stress axis dysfunction.

CHILDHOOD ADVERSITY AND STRESS RESPONSES

Research shows that children who experience sexual, physical and emotional maltreatment, domestic violence, parental loss and separation, or neglect are prone to the development of physical health issues due to a dysregulated HPA axis. These health disorders include a higher prevalence of autoimmune diseases,[1] obesity,[2] cardiovascular disease[3] and dramatically accelerated biological ageing.[4]

However, it is in the mental health domain that the greatest vulnerabilities exist. In a large study looking at childhood adversity with associations to mental health disorders (depression, anxiety disruptive behaviour and substance abuse), Harvard researchers found that 44.6 per cent of childhood and 32 per cent of adult onset mental health issues can be attributed to childhood adversity.[5]

STRESS AXIS REGULATION – IT'S EASIER THAN WE REALISE

Regaining control over the stress axis and dysregulated cortisol is important when looking to promote resilience. Fortunately, there are several ways to successfully achieve this, which include breathing exercises, strengthening relationships, nutritional supplements and dietary interventions, pharmaceutical agents, specific forms of exercise and activity, spending time in nature and lifestyle choices. Remarkably, of the many strategies to choose from (including medication), social support and human connection shine the brightest.

Take a moment to reflect on a time when you experienced a stressful event that really unsettled you and no matter how hard you tried, or how many deep breaths you took, you just couldn't settle or self-soothe. And then someone close to you (a parent, partner or very close friend) walks into the room, your eyes connect and you immediately feel calmer and more secure. Their presence hasn't necessarily removed the stressor or changed the external circumstances, but unbeknown to you it has influenced your biological and emotional state without a word of advice dispensed or any comfort given.

SOCIAL BUFFERING

According to Megan Gunner from the Institute of Childhood Development at the University of Minnesota, what I have just described is a subset of social support known as social buffering. It is one of the most powerful ways to modulate stress perceptions and responses.[6]

During early childhood, parents are the primary stress regulators for children, although a child's temperament (i.e. extroversion, openness, consciousness and agreeableness) and their genetic make-up interact with parenting quality to predict their responses to fear, pain, trauma and uncertainty.

Parental support remains a potent stress buffer into late childhood, but it begins to lose its effectiveness by adolescence (10–19 years), something that every parent has to come to (sometimes reluctantly) accept. Puberty and its associated hormonal changes appears to be the major switch that alters the potency of parental buffering. During this stage of life friends tend to serve as primary stress buffers, especially when social dynamics are the source of stress, which is often the case in those adolescent years. By adulthood, husbands, wives, life partners or very close friends assume this protective and critically supportive role.

The mechanism behind the profound effect of having supportive people in our lives and their role in buffering stress is not fully understood. However, what research has revealed is that there are at least two primary drivers in reduced stress axis activation and lower cortisol responses to adversity. The first influence emanates from brain behaviour and regional activation patterns.[7] Neuroimaging studies show that the mere presence of a close companion or family member reduces activity in the areas of the brain that process stress, fear, threat and pain. At the same time, the executive regions light up, showing cognitive control and authority over negative emotional experiences.

A simple analogy is to see our brain and its collection of distinct regions as individuals who make up a rugby team (or any team sport). In this team, each player has a specific position and key role to play. Under normal game conditions and against a weaker opponent, the team operates in total harmony, with every member understanding and fulfilling their respective roles and responsibilities. However, in adversity and under more stressful conditions, there are some players who are prone to basic errors, while there are others who simply thrive under such conditions. The emotional centres in our brain are those players who tend to "fumble the ball" and miss those all-important tackles, whereas the brain's executive regions are the "impact" players who soak up the pressure with relative ease. The stronger and more trained these impact players are (i.e. the better they engage, the more connected they are to the emotional circuits), and the more the team relies on them in challenging and pressurised situations, the better everyone's overall performance and outcomes. In other words, resilience demands that intellect prevails over emotion.

While we don't need science to affirm what we intuitively know, which is that having special people in our lives acts as safety cues that ultimately reorganise brain activity in favour of resilience and stress tolerance, it is certainly a nice validation. Perhaps this affirmation will nudge us to make a greater effort in reconnecting with those people we have lost touch with due to the social changes brought on by the pandemic in 2020. Or alternatively, it can serve as a strong reminder of the immense value that people hold in our lives and motivates us to show them more gratitude, appreciation and care.

Sadly, there are many people around the world who don't have people in their lives who provide social buffering, let alone provide other forms of support during difficult periods. This stark reality exists for one-third of the world's population who are currently experiencing considerable loneliness[8] (the discrepancy between our desired and our actual social relationships). Most of us would assume that COVID-19 is largely to blame for this existing global phenomenon. While it has dramatically amplified the burden, the loneliness crisis has been a global burden for some time. In 2018 the UK appointed the world's first minister for loneliness.[9]

The pressing question is how can we promote resilience and optimise brain activity and recruitment patterns when social support is lacking or non-existent? Fortunately, it is possible and very attainable with a little work and focused effort. Although human connection is something we should all strive for, the strongest alternative to social support and human connection is mindfulness meditation. Mindfulness is essentially a practice of learning to monitor and accept things, two behaviours that are rare in our modern world.

MINDFULNESS PARALLELS SOCIAL SUPPORT IN REDUCING STRESS

Several studies show that higher levels of the trait mindfulness are associated with reduced cortisol and lower stress reactivity under adverse conditions.[10] In 2014 David Creswell, a professor of psychology from Carnegie Mellon University, published a paper that identified the core mechanisms through which mindfulness promotes resilience and reduces vulnerability.

Firstly, the practice increases the recruitment of executive regions (specifically the ventral and dorsal regions of the lateral prefrontal cortex) of the brain, which can indirectly reduce activity in stress processing areas.[11] What Creswell and his team also discovered was that mindfulness directly reduces reactivity of the central stress processing regions (amygdala, anterior cingulate cortex, hypothalamus). In other words, developing greater mindfulness will protect against obstacles, challenges, change, uncertainty, conflict or other major stressors from translating into mental and emotional vulnerability.

Moreover, neuroimaging studies dating back to 2013 have found that mindfulness not only alters function and activity of the brain's fear centre, but it also changes its entire structure.[12] If all these findings have not already convinced you as to the value and merits of mindfulness, then perhaps the fact that this form of meditation reduces connectivity of the stress processing centres within the brain might. The effect of this structural adaptation would be the reduced capacity to become emotionally incited by stress.

The lesson that can be taken from the research is that while social support is invaluable in helping us navigate life's ups and downs, mindfulness comes in a very close second.

OXYTOCIN, SOCIAL SUPPORT AND RESILIENCE

Another major benefit and subsequent influence of social buffering and human support relates to the increased expression of the neurochemical and hormone known as oxytocin. Oxytocin's impact on resilience and human performance is so profound that to date there are over 27,700 published articles on its immense and complex biological role.

This sophisticated protein, known best for its role in sex, love and affection, interacts with the who's who of human neurochemistry (cortisol, acetylcholine, GABA, glutamate, opioids, cannabinoids, catecholamines, indoleamines and sex hormones) and has a profound effect on our immune system and antioxidant defences.[13]

What the enormous body of research distinctly shows is that oxytocin helps us to cope better under stressful and challenging situations and supports physical healing and recovery.

This ancient neuropeptide (large protein) has been central to human survival from the beginning of history, largely by means of helping us to better recognise social and sensory cues and organising our physiological responses and behaviour.[14] Basically, oxytocin tells us what is going on in our immediate environment, who the influencers are and then organises the ideal physical, emotional and behavioural responses.

From a stress perspective, oxytocin is the undisputed heavyweight champion as it has the power and influence to inhibit the brain's fear and anxiety centre.[15] It can reduce cortisol release,[16] lower blood pressure and resting heart rate, and improve heart rate variability (HRV).[17] Incidentally, HRV happens to be a critical measure, reflecting levels of stress as well as psychosocial and physical health. Essentially, HRV measures the body's ability to rapidly and effectivity adjust its responses (cardiovascular, immune, hormonal) to the world around us.

Oxytocin can also take the sting out of emotional events in that it diminishes connectivity between the amygdala (fear centre) and the brain stem, the most basic and primitive portion of the human brain.[18] What this means is that our typical reaction to stressors, such as a pounding heart, sweaty palms, sleeplessness and shallow and rapid breathing, will be significantly reduced.

A multinational study found that oxytocin significantly increased connectivity between the amygdala and prefrontal cortex, offering improved potential for social cognition and emotional regulation during the most difficult of periods.[19]

With such a profound influence on our health, wellbeing and coping mechanisms, it does beg the question – what happens if we don't have social connections that can bolster and augment this neuropeptide?

Much like our neurocircuitry, there are several lifestyle activities, foods and nutritional supplements that can support the oxytocin system and, by doing so, our resilience. Nutritionally, quercetin, vitamin D, magnesium and the probiotic strain Lactobacillus reuteri are some of the stronger nutraceutical influences.

■ Quercetin

The COVID-19 pandemic made quercetin a household name due to its anti-inflammatory, antioxidant and analgesic effects. It turns out that this plant extract superhero also positively influences the oxytocin system.[20] You can increase your intake of quercetin through diet (although I am not entirely sure that you would feel an appreciable difference), and some of the best sources include cherries, apples, honey, raspberries, red grapes, citrus fruits, green leafy vegetables and onions. Alternatively, I would suggest supplementation, which can be taken at intakes of 1.1–2.3 grams per day.[21]

■ Vitamin D

Few nutrients pack the biological punch of vitamin D, including its ability to regulate oxytocin.[22] According to Dr Michael Horlick, a professor at Boston University School of Medicine who has authored over 400 publications on the benefits of vitamin D, it influences more than 80 metabolic processes (including immune function, calcium absorption, prevention of oxidative stress, mitochondrial function, neurochemical balance and many others). Additionally, Horlick attributes vitamin D to the control of almost 2,000 genes, many of which control cell growth, immune function, blood sugar stabilisation and proper brain, heart and muscle function.

Historically, most of our vitamin D would be derived from direct sunlight, but due to changes in the way we live and work, together with some of the risks associated with excessive sun exposure, many people are deficient in this vital vitamin. The supplement vitamin D3 (cholecalciferol) is recommended over D2 supplementation (ergocalciferol). The reason for this is that D3 is used more effectively in the body.

Establishing the optimal dosage of this vitamin has been a challenge to scientists for some time. Currently, the Tolerable Upper Intake Level is 4,000 IU (international units) per day, but evidence does suggest that the less conservative Tolerable Upper Intake Level is much higher, at around 10,000 IU per day.[23] If you are not experiencing any form of deficiency as established by bloodwork, then 1,000–2,000 IU per day should be sufficient. In the case of an existing vitamin D deficiency, a dose of 4,000 IU per day is recommended.

■ Lactobacillus reuteri

There has been tremendous interest in the influence of gut microbial communities and human health in recent years. A 2013 study carried out by researchers from Massachusetts Institute of Technology discovered that ingesting Lactobacillus reuteri resulted in a profound upregulation of oxytocin activity and a plethora of associated health benefits.[24]

This particular study assessed the speed of wound healing and relationship to this specific probiotic strain in mice. As we now know, healing and immune system regulation falls within the scope of oxytocin's large biological portfolio, so any improvement in wound healing would correlate to changes to the expression of this neuropeptide. The study found that by supplementing with Lactobacillus reuteri, the speed of wound healing and recovery from tissue damage was twice as fast. The researchers were also able to identify the mechanism through which this bacterial strain was able to influence neurochemistry. What they uncovered was that this bacterial species used the vagus nerve to create a high speed and real-time communication corridor between the brain and the digestive tract.

The vagus nerve is one of the longest and most influential nerves in the body. It exits the skull just behind the ears and descends vertically along the front of the throat through the chest cavity and continues down into the abdomen. It is the direct interface between the brain and key organs and systems of the body, most notably the digestive tract, heart and lungs. This so-called "wandering" nerve operates far below the level of our conscious minds. Although its primary role is synchronicity between the body and the brain, its best recognised attribute is that of calming the body following the fight-or-flight state induced by norepinephrine and epinephrine. The release of oxytocin contributes to this profound biological influence.

The best strains for supplementation include Lactobacillus reuteri ATCC 55730, DSM 17938 and ATCC 6475, as they are all known to survive oral supplementation without degradation.[25] In other words, these strains survive the digestive process whereas others may not.

Suggested doses of Lactobacillus reuteri are in the range of 1 billion to 100 billion colony-forming units (CFU) taken over the course of a day. Both single doses and multiple split doses per day have been found to be effective.

Nutritional support for oxytocin

Nutrient	Suggested dose	Goes well with	Reasons not to take
Quercetin	1.1–2.3 grams/day	Green tea or green tea extracts and resveratrol	Genetic polymorphisms in the COMT gene (under-expression)
Vitamin D	2,000–4,000 IU/day	–	Spending lengthy periods of time outdoors during the summer months
Lactobacillus reuteri	1–100 billion CFU/day	–	–
Magnesium L-threonate or glycinate	200–400 mg/day	Meals	–
Vitamin C	100–2,000 mg/day	–	Kidney stones or renal disease

SECTION SUMMARY

- The stress response causes the body to undergo large-scale reorganisation, which, if sustained, can be extremely taxing and potentially damaging emotionally, physically and mentally.
- Children who have experienced sexual, physical and emotional maltreatment, domestic violence, parental separation or significant uncertainty are predisposed to significant stress axis dysregulation, often leading to chronically elevated cortisol.
- Childhood adversity plays a significant role in the development of mental health disorders in adulthood.

- Social support is immeasurably powerful in stress regulation, as it positively influences brain activity and neurochemistry.
- Social buffering (a subset of social support) is associated with reduced activity in the brain region associated with fear, stress, threat and pain (the amygdala).
- Social buffering increases activity in the brain's executive regions (the prefrontal cortex).
- If you are experiencing loneliness, feel isolated and are struggling to manage your stress, mindfulness meditation can serve as a sound substitute to human connection, as it influences the brain in much the same way as human support and connection.
- Oxytocin is a neurochemical and hormone that drives many of the resilience and health benefits attributed to social buffering and human support.
- Oxytocin is highly influential in driving our behaviours, as it interacts with many other neurochemicals and hormones, which include cortisol, acetylcholine, GABA, glutamate, opioids, cannabinoids, catecholamines, indoleamines and sex hormones.
- Without ongoing social support, we would have to consciously augment our oxytocin system. This can be achieved through nutritional interventions, which include quercetin, vitamin D, a high-quality probiotic, magnesium and vitamin C.

LESSON 7

THE IMMUNE SYSTEM
DETERMINES OUR RESILIENCE

Early-life adversity and ongoing stress is commonly associated with hormonal and neurochemical dysregulation, which includes chronically raised levels of epinephrine and norepinephrine, together with a decline in acetylcholine (a chemical messenger that has many important brain and body functions like attention, learning, memory, movement and sleep).[1] This physiological response, which can be likened to an infection, chronic disease or even alterations to the lining of the digestive tract (intestinal permeability), results in an increase in the release of small proteins, known as cytokines, that strongly influence the degree of immune activity (i.e. regulates inflammation), both within our body and in our brain.

One of the primary mechanisms for increased brain inflammation (neuro-inflammation), as a consequence of chronic stress and adversity, is a reduction in the expression of claudin-5 within as little as ten days.[2] Claudin-5 is a protein that determines the sealing properties of the blood–brain barrier, a protective network of blood vessels and tissues that keeps many harmful substances from entering the brain. Adversity-induced reductions in claudin-5 expression creates an environment where a far greater number of blood-borne proinflammatory cytokines (most notably IL-6) cross this important barrier and enter the brain, further amplifying an already elevated intrinsic immune response, as a result of raised epinephrine and norepinephrine.[3]

The impact of neuroinflammation on resilience is profound, as heightened or dysregulated immune activity alters many important functions and processes within the brain. For example, neuroinflammation disrupts serotonin synthesis, which impacts mood, sleep, learning, cognitive flexibility and emotional behaviours. It also lowers dopamine, affecting motivation, focus and attention.[4] Raised immune activity will result in general illness symptoms, such as fatigue, loss of appetite, weakness and pain. Neuroinflammation also results in a toxic build-up of metabolic by-products (most notably quinolinic acid), which causes the increased expression of glutamate, a neurochemical that can cause significant nerve damage in excess. In addition, it changes the function of cortisol from an anti-inflammatory hormone to a proinflammatory trigger and causes the reduced formation of new brain cells in key regions, largely by lowered expression of BDNF.

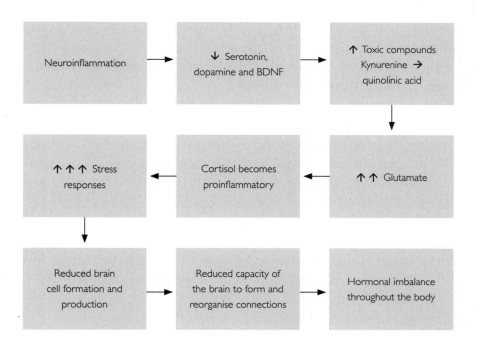

In other words, neuroinflammation is associated with reduced brain cell formation (neurogenesis), impaired connectivity (neuroplasticity), heightened stress reactivity and a significant degree of neurochemical and hormonal imbalance. Even without understanding the science and these intricate biological details, we have all experienced this emotionally, mentally and physically compromised state at various points in our life when stress has been overwhelming and sustained. The question we must be asking is why does the body respond to adversity in this seemingly odd and counterintuitive way?

NEUROINFLAMMATION IS A SOPHISTICATED DEFENCE

As extreme as this adversity-mediated adaptation may appear, it is not a physiological glitch or shortcoming but rather a remarkably sophisticated short-term defence mechanism. Essentially, neuroinflammation promotes a greater sensitivity to negative or threatening experiences, helping us to circumnavigate them more effectively.

At the same time, the raised immune activity within our brain makes us far more receptive to positive social experiences, driving us towards connection and promoting the reinforcement of close relationships, which in turn lowers the experience of vulnerability.

Think about the last time you had a cold or flu and your immune system was in overdrive. In the midst of the experience, when you were feeling your worst, your natural instinct was probably to disconnect and withdraw from the outside world. At the same time, our most basic instincts will draw us closer to our immediate circle of family and friends, as they are the ones who care for us in moments of vulnerability and physical fragility.

However, this short-term defence (a few days at most) is not well adapted to the extreme adversity and chronic stress that we experience in this day and age. Perpetual neuroinflammation will neither support functional adaptability nor structural neuroplasticity, which are both critical in the development of long-term resilience.

■

INFLAMMATION PUTS THE BRAKES ON RECOVERY

Recovery and the capacity to bounce back from setbacks, both emotionally and physically, are also key factors in resilience. At the core of the human recovery experience is immune system integrity and regulation. Research in the areas of physical trauma and mental health compromise show that protracted inflammation (for months or years on end) impairs recovery from affected states, with negative consequences within the framework of resilience and successful adaptation.[5 6]

■

DEPRESSION AND ANXIETY HAVE IMMUNE SYSTEM TIES

In light of the understanding that neuroinflammation reduces dopamine, serotonin and BDNF, it should come as no surprise to learn that chronically raised immune markers, such as C-reactive protein (CRP), Tumor necrosis factor alpha (TNF-α) and most notably IL-6, are strongly associated with depression.[7] In many respects, this knowledge and understanding can be empowering, and having regular blood work done can offer an objective and measurable window into your existing emotional state and level of progress through various interventions (pharmaceutical, behavioural or lifestyle).

Additionally, childhood maltreatment and/or difficult socio-economic circumstances in the formative years are both linked to chronic inflammation in adult life, increasing the risk and susceptibility to post-traumatic stress disorder (PTSD).[8]

PTSD often presents many years following adversity and traumatic events. According to the Mayo Clinic, symptoms of PTSD include intrusive memories (reliving the event, upsetting dreams, severe physical or emotional reactions to reminders), avoidance (places, people and thoughts that act as reminders), negative changes to thought patterns and mood (detachment, lack of interest, negative perceptions, numbness and hopelessness) and changes to physical or emotional reactions (being easily frightened, being permanently on guard, self-destructive behaviour such as substance abuse, binge eating, gambling, sleep disorders and frequent emotional outbursts).[9]

While chronic inflammation is associated with PTSD, it is also linked to other forms of anxiety. In a review entitled "Inflammation in Fear- and Anxiety-Based Disorders: PTSD, GAD, and Beyond", researchers from Harvard and Emory universities identified that all forms of fear responses and anxiety, whether generalised anxiety, phobias (social, agoraphobia, etc.) or panic disorders, may emanate from chronic inflammation.[10]

■
RESILIENCE HAS A BIOMARKER

By contrast, research shows that resilient individuals of all ages show lower inflammatory markers and greater immune regulation overall.[11] There is growing evidence that low or lower levels of IL-6 are a robust biomarker for resilience across all age groups.[12]

There are many risk factors that contribute to neuroinflammation and subsequent vulnerability to challenge and adversity. These include chronic stress and repeated trauma in childhood, an ongoing absence of social support and human connection, poor diet and lifestyle, environmental pollution, infections and chronic diseases, inherited genetic variants in the inflammatory cytokine genes (specifically IL-6) or alternatively under-expression (due to genetic factors) of anti-inflammatory cytokines (specifically IL-10).

■

IT'S A MINDSET

Despite the immense complexity that exists within the immune system and its relationship to resilience, like with so many of the previously discussed resilience-promoting strategies, improved regulation is achievable, no matter how compromised we are or how chronic and extreme our experience of adversity and stress has been during our lives.

Although our knee-jerk reaction would be to explore medications and nutritional supplements as a first-line support tool, the immune-modulating journey needs to begin with our intrinsic behaviours and the way we perceive and interact with the world around us. The reality is that psychological coping strategies have a profound effect on immune regulation (without any long-term side effects), largely through buffering stress and challenge.

Personal control, positive affect and optimism are some of these numerous coping strategies available to us.

Exercise personal control

Studies have shown that the belief that you can achieve set goals and control your life's destination, no matter the circumstances, is a strong predictor of resilience.[13] One of the greatest minds of our time, the late Lord Rabbi Doctor Jonathan Sacks, was able to communicate this principle so eloquently in his book *Morality: Restoring the Common Good in Divided Times*.

Lord Sacks, a recipient of 16 honorary degrees, believed that we face two choices when confronted with hardship, challenges and pain.

The first choice is that we live and experience the situation as an object that has little power or authority over the events that are unfolding. For example, the COVID-19 pandemic brought significant financial challenges, loneliness and social isolation, personal loss and grief and an immense degree of uncertainty about the future in all areas of life.

The feeling that we are being acted upon by uncontrollable forces far greater than ourselves, and the associated helplessness, manifests in strong negative emotions that include anger, bitterness, resentment and blame. Any goals we may have had are often replaced with the desire to simply survive the event itself. We can all identify in some way with this at some point in our lives.

However, Sacks describes an alternative mindset that takes the focus away from "Why did this happen?", "Why me?" and "Why now?" to a more resilient dialogue of "What shall I do?" The moment we look forward as opposed to backward, we choose to become a subject (as opposed to an object), giving us more authority over our life path and ultimately our destination. With this mindset, the realisation of goals once again becomes a central aspect of our life journey.

Making the decision to think and act in a future-orientated manner isn't easy; in fact, it is anything but! This may explain why many people remain locked in a personal comfort zone of anger and bitterness. This important choice, which culminates in ultimate success, requires you to face your challenges directly (as opposed to withdrawing), the courage to change, the bravery to fail, the strength to stand up time and time again after being knocked down and the self-control to keep on the journey and not revert to self-sabotage. As difficult as this may appear, the reality is that the world has undergone, and is still undergoing, profound changes on political, social and economic fronts. If we wish to realise our dreams and aspirations amid these exponential changes, we simply *have* to look forward and train ourselves to continue doing so.

When we practise self-dialogue, continually reinforcing "I can do anything I set my mind to" and above that set clear and short-, medium- and long-term goals, we become the pilot of our own destiny. Remarkably, this simple shift in self-belief creates greater stability and regulation within our immune system.

A 2017 study by researchers from the University of Rochester on 4,779 older individuals with higher perceived levels of personal control (I am a subject, I chose my life path and destination) showed that, regardless of their health or lifetime traumatic experiences, inflammatory markers were lower than those who had higher levels of perceived constraints (what happens to me is beyond my control), supporting greater resilience and providing significant health protection.[14]

Positive emotions

Feelings of love, gratitude, joy, serenity, inspiration, enthusiasm, humour, accomplishment and so on have been shown to promote a significant degree of immune regulation and overall resilience. There are many theories as to the mechanism through which these positive emotions translate to better mental, emotional and physical health. Some researchers have suggested that that positive influence is due to the body's opioid (endorphins), oxytocin, norepinephrine, dopamine and serotonin systems being upregulated, which is in itself a strong counterweight to negativity. Or alternatively, positive emotions generate broader perspectives, bigger-picture thinking, creative problem-solving and encourage many restorative activities, such as better sleep, exercise, relaxation (meditation, massage, yoga), family holidays, social connection and spending time in nature.

Positive emotions are associated with better health, less pain and even greater life expectancy.[15] Think back to a time when you were chronically stressed and felt burnt out, and in the nick of time you were able to get away to a remote location. At the time of your departure, you might have been feeling a bit sick or run-down, possibly congested with a runny nose and aching body. However, this was completely overshadowed by the experience of extreme exhaustion and general discomfort (bloating, puffiness, agitation). The travel day was probably the most challenging of all, with last-minute work to finish and the complexities of packing, cars and perhaps even flying. But once you do arrive at your destination, it is worth the monumental effort.

The next morning you wake up still feeling tired and exhausted, but happy. The view is spectacular, the air is clean and it's quiet and peaceful. You wonder to yourself why you don't do this more often, as you feel so relaxed. The honest answer is that it is really expensive and time availability doesn't always allow for frequent breaks, but you tell yourself that it is simply a matter of bad scheduling or poor self-management and you commit to make a lifestyle change, favouring frequent breaks. As the day progresses, you feel happier and more content. Your health and wellbeing exponentially improve and fatigue, congestion and physical pain give way to excitement, enthusiasm and curiosity. Within less than 48 hours, your health is given a much-needed reset – both emotionally and physically.

There are many examples of positive experiences (i.e. a new relationship, future opportunity, being inspired by a person or event, etc.) providing a vehicle for the reduced experience of vulnerability in adversity. We cannot underestimate the power and influence that joy, happiness, excitement, contentment, gratitude and enthusiasm have on our overall wellbeing.

A large study done by researchers from the University of California, involving 150,048 individuals from 142 countries, found that positive emotions were more predictive of long-term health than basic needs, such as the availability of food, shelter and safety.[16] This was found to be more notable in disadvantaged communities.

Living in a country where inequality and poverty is so prevalent and human pain and suffering so overt, it might be hard to get your head around this finding; but the point is abundantly clear, do not underestimate the power of positivity in the human experience.

How do we even begin to be positive when it feels like the weight of the world is on our shoulders? It begins with a conscious decision to take the time to acknowledge what we have as opposed to what we don't. Perhaps it is creating moments of serenity in the day when you listen to enjoyable music or get outside into nature for a break. It could be exploring new interests or showing greater love and affection to the special people in your life. In truth, there are countless ways we are able to experience positive emotions and science has also provided some simple and effective hacks.

Research going back several decades has shown that positive emotions following stressful events, and even spontaneous smiling during emotional experiences, helps the cardiovascular system to recover faster and supports biological stability and more regulated immune behaviours. Also, periods of happiness occurring alongside anxiety completely counteract the profound blood pressure changes seen in distressed states.[17]

This can be applied to our lives in a number of ways:

- If you plan on watching TV after a stressful day, watch a comedy or light-hearted series that will make you laugh and smile, as opposed to a thriller or drama that can trigger arousal, stress, anxiety and/or fear.
- When placed in a stressful situation, such as a pressurised meeting, presentation or interview, it can be helpful to try to smile more, thereby assisting in regulating your stress axis.
- Make an extra effort to do something you really enjoy during the more stressful periods of your life. Whether it be daily, weekly or at the very least monthly, the experience of happiness, enthusiasm and contentment is transformative and supportive in the broader resilience framework.

Optimism, optimism, optimism

Optimism reflects the extent to which you believe your future is going to be positive. Optimism often gets confused with toxic positivity, which is an obsession with positive thinking (not to be mistaken for positive emotions). Toxic positivity is the belief that you have to put a positive spin on every event, regardless of the experience of challenge, pain or hurt. While the intention is to silence negative emotions (which can be noble), it can be construed as demeaning and insensitive to others who are going through their own hardships and it places external pressure on people to withhold their true feelings and emotions. This pattern of behaviour dates back to the late 1990s and the establishment of the positive psychology movement.

Toxic positivity was alive and well during the initial waves of the COVID-19 pandemic, specifically during the lockdowns. One morning Jess, a close friend, confided in my wife that the boutique hotel that her husband owned had folded due to the many prohibitions within the hospitality industry. He simply didn't have the financial reserves to hold out for the initially forecast three months. My wife was sobbing, his wife was sobbing. "What can we do to help?" my wife asked me. I immediately picked up the phone (I would have driven there if I had been allowed to) to offer my support (emotional, instrumental, financial) to Jess's husband, Mike. When Mike answered my call, I looked at my screen to see if I called the right number – he was incredibly upbeat, stating that happiness is a choice and he just needed to pivot things in his life. In an attempt to be sensitive, I didn't feel it was my place to move the conversation to Mike's business and personal challenges. Over the next few weeks of lockdown, Mike continued to brush off his problems, hide his true feelings and hold his reality very close to his chest. When the COVID-19 restrictions finally lifted, and we were able to meet up in person, Mike's experiences had taken their toll on his health, physical appearance and overall demeanour. Fortunately, Mike was able to find new opportunities and is currently doing extremely well.

Mike and Jess reflect what many people went through in 2020. Countless families went through similar painful experiences and the conversations followed a similar pattern: because of social and societal norms, we no longer feel secure enough to express our vulnerability. The net effect is a suppression of the entire experience through the silencing of negative emotions.

Optimism differs from toxic positivity in that it doesn't dismiss or diminish the current hardships, hurdles, personal struggle and pain, but rather accepts the need to acknowledge and recognise them. At the same time, optimism is the strong belief that the future will be better and that we have the ability to influence the direction of our life through the decisions we make and the choices we take.

Hope

In 2010 researchers from several prominent US universities published a study on the relationship between optimism, pessimism and immune activity. The study was large and involved 6,814 participants, aged 45–84, and investigated a personal inherent level of optimism or pessimism in relation to cardiovascular disease. The researchers were specifically monitoring the major immune factors, such as IL-1, IL-6 and CRP as well as many clotting and health markers, such as fibrinogen (a protein that is essential for clot formation) and homocysteine (a protein that is a risk factor in cardiovascular disease).[18]

The researchers found that optimism, as measured by the Revised Life Orientation Test (LOT-R), a 10-item scale developed by Michael Scheier at Carnegie Mellon University, was associated with considerably lower levels of IL-6 and CRP and other major health markers. Conversely, pessimism and negativity were associated with raised inflammatory markers to the extent that it reflected a 10-year increase in biological age. In other words, negativity ages you!

How does optimism translate into better immune functionality and health? The power in believing that the future will be better and that our dreams will be realised transcends our emotional and mental state into the realm of action. When we are optimistic about the future, we tend to build and align habits and behaviours that support a positive reality. It is the combined effect of the belief in a better future, positive habits and actions that ultimately promotes better health and resilience. Supporting this assertion, a Dutch study found that intrinsic optimism was associated with better self care that encompassed more physical activity, higher intakes of healthy food and other positive lifestyle habits.[19] At the same time, evidence shows that optimism impacts the stress axis by reducing cortisol and lowering blood pressure[20] and is associated with accelerated recovery from challenges and adversity. If any of these influences are sounding vaguely familiar as a collective set, it is because a central driver in favourable future expectations happens to be the neuropeptide oxytocin. A genetic study done at the University of California found that not only is oxytocin a driver of optimism and greater self-esteem but also of personal control (mastery).[21]

This is a significant insight. The value in understanding the underlying molecular driver in optimism, personal control and positive emotions is such that should we experience barriers in these areas, the opportunity to move forward may be through improving the expression and uptake of oxytocin.

We have all experienced moments when the challenges appear too great or the personal pain is all-consuming. Despite a deeper understanding of the value and future implications of shifting our thinking into a positive state, we are simply unable to and feel powerless in the moment.

Instead of attempting to suppress our immediate experience, or wrestling with conflicting emotions, we can approach our experience with a bit of distance and self-compassion. Oxytocin is an immensely powerful protein that has the potential to shift the trajectory of how we feel and think. By taking on habits and behaviours that support the expression and utilisation of this neuropeptide (I have already provided nutritional levers and will be discussing the social and physical drivers later in the book) we are able to slowly reignite and reengage positive emotions, personal control and optimism.

SECTION SUMMARY

- Chronically raised levels of epinephrine and norepinephrine typically accompany adversity.
- Adversity causes a greater influx of proinflammatory cytokines to enter the brain, resulting in a significant and adverse immune reaction.
- Brain inflammation disrupts serotonin production, lowers dopamine and decreases BDNF expression. This has a negative impact on mental and emotional health as well as cognitive performance.
- Neuroinflammation inhibits new brain cell formation, impairs regional connectivity, heightens stress reactivity and impairs stress axis regulation.
- In the short term, neuroinflammation can be a powerful defence mechanism, as it makes us more sensitive to negative or threatening situations, helping us to avoid them more effectively.
- Vulnerability as a consequence of neuroinflammation makes us more receptive to positive social experiences and pushes us towards connection and social support.
- While short-lived inflammation can and does offer various protections, chronic inflammation significantly impairs brain structure and function, reducing long-term adaptability and overall resilience.
- Depression and anxiety are highly correlated with elevated immune markers, including CRP, TNF-α and IL-6.
- Lower levels of the immune marker IL-6 are associated with improved resilience.
- Our perspective and behaviours have a profound influence on immune behaviours, more so than we realise.
- The perception of personal control, positive emotions and optimism are all associated with lower inflammatory markers and improved immune regulation.

LESSON 8

THE HEALTH BEHAVIOURS THAT SHAPE OUR REALITY

Many health behaviours, such as good nutrition, exercise and a healthy lifestyle, can exert a positive and regulatory effect on IL-6 and subsequently enhance resilience. However, it is important to mention the behaviours that elevate IL-6 and that result in increased inflammation and greater overall vulnerability to adversity and stress. Some of these triggers include excessive alcohol intake (whereas moderate consumption may confer benefit),[1] sleep deprivation (causing a three-fold increase in IL-6 expression),[2] high consumption of processed sugar (especially during puberty)[3][4] and smoking.[5] This means that in order to improve your resilience many of these habits need to be managed more carefully.

■

THE HABITS THAT DEFINE US

Without health, we have nothing. The value of health practices in chronic disease prevention and life extension are well established. However, it is only in the last decade or so that the value of health behaviours in the promotion of resilience and mental wellbeing has been fully appreciated. This new understanding stems from research done in elite military circles, where numerous studies have identified that soldier resilience (measured under some of the most testing and harsh conditions) is strongly correlated to greater physical health, higher levels of fitness and overall physical preparedness, which in turn positively influences psychological factors, such as stress regulation, emotional and cognitive control, self-confidence, effective goal setting, etc.[6]

Health promotion practices fall under a broad canopy, but they can be categorised into primary areas. (Although the environment and behaviours are also strong contributing factors):

- Exercise and physical activities
- Dietary practices and nutrition

These parts can be independently and collectively used to promote adaptability, effect structural changes in the brain, aid in neuroplasticity and enhance performance across all areas of our life.

■

MOVE!

There are many reasons why exercise and physical activity should form the backbone of any resilience programme. One of the primary benefits of regular exercise is radically improved performance (i.e. in the expression, transportation or uptake) of dopamine, norepinephrine and serotonin[7] – key neurochemicals that govern our mental and emotional wellbeing. These molecules support our mental health as well as overall human performance and the actualisation of potential through enhanced motivation, drive and cognition. Exercise (even a single session) is also associated with a dramatic increase in BDNF,[8] thereby reinforcing neuroplasticity and adaptability and in turn bolstering resilience.

The neurochemical shifts that occur during and after exercise can negate and even reverse negative changes that occur within the brain as a consequence of neuroinflammation and chronic stress. Astoundingly, physical activity doesn't just alter our neurochemical state; it also positively affects our immune system, which is why exercise offers an unmatched protection against vulnerability in response to adversity.

The effect of exercise on immune behaviours has only recently been understood, although researchers admit there is so much more to be learnt. What *is* known is that exercise doesn't necessarily lead to reduced expression of IL-6 (in fact, forceful muscle contractions elevate IL-6), but the positive immune effects seen in the brain and periphery occur due to a robust and protracted spike in at least eight anti-inflammatory factors, most notability IL-10 and BDNF.[9] The research also shows that the more you exercise over the course of your lifetime, the greater the production and release of these anti-inflammatory agents.[10]

For decades, research has consistently shown that ageing and adversity have much in common in that they both alter immune signalling and, as a consequence, promote a proinflammatory internal environment.[11]

A 2020 study published in the *Journal of Applied Physiology* sought to answer the question as to whether or not an increase in low-grade inflammation could be positivity influenced by regular exercise throughout our lifespan. The academics compared 10 young and healthy exercisers, 10 older and healthy non-exercisers and 21 lifelong exercisers with over 50 years of consistent training activity who were all free from disease and injuries and were non-smokers.[12]

Consistent training activity was defined as either running or cycling five times a week for approximately seven hours in total. The analysis used both blood inflammatory markers (specifically C-reactive protein, IL-6, TNF-α and IGF-1) at rest and muscle biopsies of the thigh muscle (a rather unpleasant procedure) before and after an exercise challenge.

The muscle biopsy aimed to examine how their muscles were adapting to physical stress from an immune and genetic perspective. The results were astounding.

The first significant finding was that at rest, lifelong exercisers had much lower levels of IL-6 (almost 50 per cent lower) than non-exercisers. Also, lifelong exercisers had a greater expression of the anti-inflammatory molecule IL-10 than non-exercisers (more than 43 per cent). The study confirmed what fitness enthusiasts intuitively know – lifelong exercise has major anti-inflammatory benefits, but added to that it could partially preserve immune behaviours seen in very young, healthy and resilient individuals. In other words, exercise is the key to our healthspan (freedom from disease across our lifetime), adaptability and future performance.

■

WHAT IS THE MOST EFFECTIVE EXERCISE FOR RESILIENCE AND IMMUNE HEALTH?

A lot of research papers have been published on what the best type of exercise is to improve resilience, and the conclusion is that it all works!

Low-intensity training (60–70 per cent of maximum heart rate [MHR]), medium-intensity training (70–80 per cent of MHR), high-intensity aerobic training (80–90 per cent of MHR), high-intensity interval training (85–95 per cent of MHR for 20 seconds up to 4 minutes), resistance training and resistance and aerobic training combined all significantly reduce IL-6 and other major inflammatory markers *in the long term* (including C-reactive protein and TNF-α), whether you are healthy, unhealthy, young or old.[13] It is important to realise that short-term exercise increases inflammation as part of the adaptive process.

Aerobic training zones

To estimate your maximum age-related heart rate, subtract your age from 220. For example, for a 45-year-old person the estimated maximum age-related heart rate would be calculated as 220 – 45 years = 175 beats per minute (bpm). To establish the high intensity zone, calculate 175 x 0.80 = 140 bpm, and 90% level would be 175 x 0.90 = 157 bpm.		
Low-intensity (zone 2)	60–70% of MHR	Sustainable for a few hours
Medium-intensity (zone 3)	71–80% of MHR	Tough to go beyond 60 minutes
High-intensity (zone 4)	81–90% of MHR	Only performed for 15–20 minutes
Very-high-intensity (zone 5)	91–100% of MHR	Only maintained for 1–2 minutes
High-intensity interval training	86–100% of MHR	For 20 seconds up to 4 minutes

The harder you work the less vulnerable you become

High-intensity interval training (HIIT) may have some distinct advantages in the promotion of resilience from an immune, hormonal, neurochemical and behavioural perspective. The distinctive advantages include: significantly reduced body fat, an unsurpassed release of BDNF (resulting in reduced anxiety, enhanced memory, greater learning capacity and even higher IQ) and strengthening of our mental capacity to withstand and overcome extreme challenges.

Lower relative body fat supports greater resilience

High-intensity interval training involves as little as three short all-out sprints of 20-40 seconds each and is associated with a sustained elevation in growth hormone (GH) that can last for over 90 minutes.[14] GH is secreted by the pituitary gland and this neuropeptide hormone has numerous biological functions, including cell reproduction and growth, supporting DNA integrity, maintaining strong bones and youthful skin, ensuring neurological integrity, promoting muscle tone and size, and optimal functioning of the cardiovascular and immune systems. Lastly, it plays a lead role in determining body composition (the level of body fat in relation to other body tissues and fluids).

What is especially relevant within the context of immune behaviours and resilience is GH's ability to reduce body fat, especially in and around the organs (i.e. visceral fat).[15] This is significant in relation to immune behaviours. At least 30 per cent of circulating IL-6 is produced by our fat cells, most notably in our visceral fat deposits.[16] Therefore, it is plausible that by reducing visceral fat through high-intensity interval training or other GH triggers, such as intermittent fasting (a topic covered extensively in my first book, *The Stress Code*), and deliberate heat exposure (i.e. sauna), not only would one experience greater overall health and vitality but also superior resilience and reduced vulnerability to adversity through the associated immune adaptations.

THE PARADOX

Strangely enough, long-term inflammation and therefore resilience is controlled and counteracted by the degree to which IL-6 is released during bouts of exercise and, in the case of HIIT, more is better!

High-intensity training of all types is associated with a robust expression of IL-6 that peaks twice – immediately post-exercise and then again one hour after. This differs from lighter physical exercise activities, such as brisk walking, hiking, jogging, swimming and cycling, which only achieve a single spike in IL-6 in the 60 minutes following the activity.[17]

Also, and most importantly, research shows that IL-6 released exclusively through muscle activation is another major stimulus in the reduction of visceral fat (by up to 20 per cent) and the prevention of its accumulation over the course of our lifetime.[18] This is good for the waistline as well as our capacity to handle challenges.

In other words, due to vastly different signalling pathways, when muscle contractions cause the release of IL-6 it supports a long-term anti-inflammatory state. By contrast, the release of IL-6 in the immune cells or visceral fat can have the opposite effect, essentially driving a chronic proinflammatory internal environment.

High intensity = high adaptability

Exercise has been shown to be a potent trigger in the release of BDNF. Research shows that increases in BDNF following exercise range from 11.7 per cent to 410 per cent, depending on individual genetic make-up, age, current state of health and the actual activity itself.[19] What has also been discovered is that BDNF expression follows a linear trajectory in relation to intensity, i.e. the harder and more physically taxing the training session, the greater the increase in BDNF.

Wishing to understand the effects of exercise on BDNF better, Swiss and Belgian scientists performed a study comparing two higher intensity aerobic exercise protocols and their respective influence on this powerful protein.[20] The comparison was over a 20-minute period when participants performed a continuous exercise protocol at 70 per cent of their maximal work rate (MWR) versus a high-intensity session at 90 per cent of their MWR for one minute, alternating with one minute of rest (i.e. ten hard efforts – not an easy undertaking).

The study revealed that BDNF levels elevate rapidly at around the 7-minute mark (although the continuous approach did result in a slightly more rapid increase) and continued to surge for the full duration of the 20-minute session.

At the same time, levels remained elevated after the session was completed. While BDNF levels showed similar peaks at around the eight-minute mark, from the tenth minute the HIIT training caused BDNF levels to take off, a trend that continued until the session was completed.

When comparing the two protocols, it was shown that continuous aerobic exercise causes a 23.7 per cent rise in BDNF over a 20-minute period, which is in itself remarkable. That said, the HIIT resulted in a staggering 37.2 per cent spike (a 35 per cent overall difference) within the same time period. Surprisingly, cortisol was 21 per cent lower with the HIIT protocol. This is surprising because the levels of cortisol in response to physical or mental exertion typically follow a very linear path. The harder and longer the activity or strain, the greater the cortisol elevation.[21] HIIT seems to offer something rather unique – high exertion with reduced cortisol responses.

From a resilience and overall human potential perspective, the benefits of raised BDNF are incalculable. For example, a mere 12 per cent increase positively effects behaviour (self-regulation, emotional expression, social skills, etc.) and a 20 per cent increase promotes new language acquisition (which could include coding, maths or even music).[22] Research shows that a 10–30 per cent spike in BDNF can dramatically improve cognition, creativity, IQ and memory. At the same time, increases in BDNF strongly protect against anxiety and depression.[23]

As impressive as these benefits are, there is an additional advantage to increased BDNF – immune modulation. In a review article titled "Physical Exercise Inhibits Inflammation and Microglial Activation", researchers from National Cheng Kung University identified that BDNF blocks several key inflammatory pathways and increases activity in anti-inflammatory genes. Additionally, the Taiwanese team believe that this super-protein may directly inhibit the brain's intrinsic immune system, known as the microglia.

Physical tolerance and resilience

When given the option, two-thirds of people choose HIIT over continuous aerobic training due to the variety that exists within the session itself and because it saves time. Yet, despite these pull factors, it is incredibly intense and will push your limits of tolerance.

There is something enthralling and confidence building about over-coming difficult physical challenges, whether they are thrown at us or are deliberate and intentional. Andrew Huberman, a highly regarded professor of neurobiology at Stanford University, views regular exposure to intense physical challenges as a key component in developing short-term stress tolerance and desensitisation.

This idea is central to the training ethos of many (if not all) special force military units throughout the world, who develop and build their teams' resilience and stress tolerance through exposure to extreme physical training and harsh environmental conditions.

I had first-hand experience of how extreme physical challenges can improve resilience when I was drafted into the South African navy in 1991 as part of a mandatory national service act. It was a tumultuous time in South Africa, with the South African Border War (involving Namibia, Zambia and Angola) ending only two years earlier and much-needed sweeping political changes taking place, which would eventually see the iconic Nelson Mandela take over the South African presidency. The military was restructuring and disbanding many of its elite units, which meant that many of the former personnel were reassigned. My basic training intake was the recipient of this restructuring.

I didn't want to be there and I certainly didn't believe in what it stood for and so I tried everything possible to get out the drafting. Because of the widespread negative views of the enforced service, the government managed to seal every conceivable exit strategy. Bar leaving the country for good, there was no perceivable way around it.

I arrived at basic training unprepared, undisciplined, emotionally and mentally vulnerable and very unfit. So unfit that a five-minute light jog would have felt like an elite-level HIIT session.

Day one was brutal and seemed to go on forever. My lungs were raw from gasping for air, my knees and back were in agony, my neck and head grazed from carrying either a bed or cupboard as part of the drill instructor's fitness vision for us, and mentally I was not coping. The next 42 days only got more intense as the elite forces' instructors attempted to expose the fragility of the human mind and body of the men within our group. Fridays were "special" in a "good luck, hope to see you at the end of the day in one piece" scenario.

I was teamed up with eight other men and we had to run, climb and crawl through a 10-kilometre obstacle course. The course involved climbing large sand dunes (we were based in Saldanha Bay), which felt as high as the Empire State building, carrying two enormous tractor tyres, steel beds (single fortunately), 25–30kg backpacks, our rifles and other random items like a steel cupboard or something equally difficult and uncomfortable to carry. Looking back, it sounds like a painful audition for a furniture removal company.

The Friday event started in the ocean doing push-ups in our full kit. The cold water was always around 12–13°c and merely added to our physical discomfort. There are only a few things that must be as painful as the combination of salt water, drenched clothing, vigorous and repetitive movement and sweat. That friction hurts, especially under the arms and between the thighs, and not just for the training exercise but for days after.

For six consecutive weeks I struggled through this Friday training exercise, largely due to having such a low base of physical fitness. Mentally and emotionally, the Friday challenge always felt unmanageable and at times too painful to bear. Also, finishing at the back of the squad didn't bode well or do me any favours within the group, as we were judged on performance as a collective. Poor performance (measured by how long it took to complete the course) had consequences, and normally meant additional physical and psychological experiences. On an individual level, to be successful in basic training demanded anonymity and at no point did one ever want to be singled out, for the same reason you didn't want to underperform as a group. The goal was to stay in the middle of the pack, avoid eye contact and appear utterly exhausted all the time, and violating any of this meant additional pain.

Going into week seven, I felt a lot fitter, which was translating into better mental and emotional coping skills. That Friday, our team was three men short, as they had gone to the sick bay, I suspect, to avoid participating. But full squad or not, we were still required to carry, drag or tow all of the specified items.

As the exercise began, a loud warning was shouted by the base commander, stating that the bottom two teams would have to repeat the event. This captured the attention of all the recruits and their squad leaders, who were required to run alongside their team for the 10 kilometres, shouting and screaming at the troops. The notion of an ultramarathon of pain was utterly terrifying. No team wanted to come last or second last and so the event became fiercely competitive as opposed to a survival exercise to complete.

That day, amid the increased pressure and challenge, I managed to be slightly in front. Driven by radically improved endurance as my fitness had finally caught up with the rest of the team and motivated to not have to repeat the event, I found mental reserves I never knew existed. What was most surprising was the fact that one of the commanding officers felt inspired to join our struggle. Apparently he was motivated by our monumental effort and supportive team dynamic. It was exactly what we needed – an additional pair of hands and his leadership in the challenge.

A few hours later, the event was finally over and, despite our reduced numbers, we had managed to place in the top three teams.

That day, we all realised that we have the inner strength and ability to overcome any challenge, whether it be mental, emotional or physical. In a strange twist, that was also the day I began to love Fridays and the physical and mental tests that came with it.

The lesson I took from that training exercise was that we are all capable of far more than we realise. In many respects, that was the purpose of being given the military activities to complete. We all have deep physical and mental reserves that can be accessed through training and building the right habits. In many ways, the direction of my life stems from my experience that day. It wasn't a feeling of pride of placing in the top three with a smaller team that motivated my journey, but rather the commanding sense of competency that I experienced through the event, due to increased endurance and stamina and how all my emotional vulnerabilities became subjugated under these conditions.

Applying this principle of physical tolerance to your own life and in your own personal context can be the defining habit that helps bring about and solidifies your future resilience. This training of physical tolerance need not be limited to exercise or physical exertion, but could also include deliberate cold exposure (which comes with its own set of resilience-promoting benefits that include raised dopamine and norepinephrine), heat exposure (i.e. sauna) or even intermittent fasting.

RUN IT BY YOUR DOCTOR

In a review of studies of cardiac rehabilitation, no adverse or other significant clinical, haemodynamic (dynamics of blood flow), electrical or biological signs of ischaemia (restricted blood flow) or arrhythmia (abnormal heart beat) events due to participation in HIIT protocols were observed, but it is imperative to consult with your doctor before engaging in routines of this nature, due to the physical strain you are placing yourself under.

EXERCISE ROUTINE IDEAS

The following HIIT routines are the ones that I use most frequently. You can do them in the pool, on an exercise bike, assault bike, rowing machine, treadmill or on the road. Existing injuries or niggles generally determine which activity I choose that day. My goal is to select an activity that will not exacerbate an underlying physical vulnerability, i.e. if you have a wrist injury, cycling or running is less likely to aggravate it whereas swimming or rowing may cause pain or discomfort. Moreover, if you are unwell, have not slept properly or feel run-down, postpone the session to a time when you feel healthy and are able to take on the challenge. There are many health monitoring devices that can provide objective (as opposed to subjective) feedback in this regard. These include wearable fitness trackers, smart watches and other biosensors.

I use an Oura Ring (and am obsessed with it), a wedding-band-like device that collects data and provides an objective measure for sleep quality, structure, duration as well as blood oxygen sensing, heart rate, HRV, body temperature, breathing frequency and other important metrics.

Routine 1
The big one
Assault bike (or a rowing machine, treadmill or stationary bike):
- 7-minute warm-up (easy pace)
- 10–15 seconds @ 90 per cent effort, followed by 50-second recovery at an easy pace
- Repeat 3 times
- 60 seconds @ 95 per cent effort, followed by 30-second recovery at an easy pace
- Repeat 4–10 times
- 5-minute cool-down (easy pace)
- 6–12-minute stretch

Routine 2
Mixing it up
Stationary bike (or rowing machine, assault bike or treadmill):
- 5–7-minute warm-up (easy pace)
- 2 minutes @ 80 per cent effort, followed by 60-second recovery
- 90 seconds @ 85 per cent effort, followed by 60-second recovery
- 60 seconds @ 90 per cent effort, followed by 60-second recovery
- 30 seconds @ 95 per cent effort, followed by 30-second recovery
- Repeat 2–3 times

Routine 3
The Murray
This is named after the former number 1 tennis player, Andy Murray, who I frequently saw performing this routine during the peak of his career in 2015 and 2016. This routine is performed on a treadmill or for swimmers in a 25/50-metre swimming pool.

On the treadmill:
- 5–8 minute light and easy warm-up (light jog)
- 40 seconds at 12–16 kilometres/hour at an incline of 2–6 at 90–100 per cent effort
- 20 seconds complete rest (step off the treadmill)
- Repeat 4–8 times
- 5–10-minute cool-down

In the swimming pool:
- 10-minute light and easy warm-up (±18–26 lengths in 25-metre pool)
- 50 metres at 90–100 per cent effort
- 20–30 seconds complete rest
- Repeat 4–10 times
- 5–10-minute cool-down

There are endless ways to achieve the resilience (physical, emotional and cognitive) benefits of HIIT. When creating your own routines, it is important to bear in mind that the high exertion intervals should be fairly short, ideally 30–90 seconds and the rest periods (which can be active or inactive) should vary from 50–100 per cent of the actual interval duration. In other words, if you sprint for a minute, your recovery should be for 30 seconds to 1 minute before repeating.

Finally, less is more. If you are looking to enhance your athletic performance, then longer and more intense routines will be more advantageous. However, when pursuing resilience, a key precept to consider is the "least amount of effort that will deliver a positive outcome". In this instance, 5–8 intervals will more than suffice.[24] [25]

A RESILIENCE-PROMOTING DIET

For any diet plan to promote resilience it needs to create an optimal state of neurochemical, hormonal and immune balance. By contrast, food choices that burden our system through ingested chemical additives, food sensitivities, the excess consumption of sugar, proteins or animal fats, or a lack of fundamental nutrients detract from our ability to adapt and successfully overcome adversity.

Inflammation is central to the development of many (if not most) chronic diseases and as a result a considerable amount of research has been done on dietary practices and eating plans that positively influence immune behaviours by reducing IL-6 and other key proinflammatory molecules. With this wealth of knowledge available, many of these learnings can be applied in our lives for the promotion of resilience.

A review study in *Advances in Nutrition* investigated many common nutritional approaches, including vegan, vegetarian, low-carbohydrate, Mediterranean and low-fat diets in controlling inflammation and overall health.[26]

Of course, there are merits and possibly even limitations to these dietary approaches, but any health plan where you are able to successfully keep your weight within healthy ranges, your body fat percentage low, your weight-to-height ratio optimal and visceral fat to a minimum will be effective in promoting resilience.[27]

The many benefits of plant-based diets

The review found tremendous support for plant-based diets in reducing systemic inflammation. A study involving 270 people between the ages of 19 and 75 compared a normal, mixed diet to a vegetarian diet (which included diary and eggs) and found that those individuals who were on a plant-based diet had a 72 per cent overall lower inflammatory profile[28] based on serum (a component of blood) concentrations of CRP.

One of the key takeaways from the study (other than that fruit and vegetables promote an anti-inflammatory state) was that there were no obese vegetarians in the study and the number of overweight individuals on a plant-based diet were approximately three times lower than those on the mixed diet. A remarkable aspect of the health-promoting properties of a vegetarian diet is how quickly the immune system can be positively influenced. Some studies show that in as little as three weeks significant health changes can take place.

In addition, the study discovered that vegetarians tend to consume more fibre than those on a mixed diet, largely due to higher overall intakes of fruit, nuts, seeds, whole grains and vegetables. Countless studies show that higher fibre intakes are negatively correlated with IL-6.[29] In other words, the more fibre in your diet, the greater your overall health and resilience potential. Some of the higher fibre foods include legumes (beans, chickpeas, lentils), vegetables (artichokes, potato, sweet potato, broccoli, winter squash and pumpkin), fruits (avocado, pear, apple, berries andd citrus), nuts and seeds (buckwheat, quinoa, almonds) and grains (bulgur, teff, oats, brown rice).

Another benefit to restricting or eliminating animal protein (specifically red meat and poultry) is an increase in the expression of a powerful resilience-promoting protein known as Neuropeptide Y (NPY).[30] NPY functions to dampen stress responses, reduce fear, anxiety and aggression and promote sleep. It has also been shown to enhance cognition and concentration under stressful conditions. In many respects, NPY can be considered as one of most influential resilience-promoting molecules.

A study done on soldiers undergoing intense survival training showed that those who had higher NPY levels were more resilient and coped better under a variety of hostile conditions.[31] The Yale study compared special forces' soldiers and ordinary soldiers and revealed that the NPY levels in the special forces group increased dramatically during the extreme physical and psychological challenges and remained elevated for almost 24 hours afterwards. This elevation promoted and supported improved adaptability, reduced stress and gave them courage. However, in the normal soldiers, especially in those who struggled mentally and emotionally with the training exercise, there was a decrease in NPY expression, which remained reduced for days following the experience, leaving them vulnerable to replaying events and disassociation behaviours.

While low (below baseline) levels of NPY can create a state of hypervigilance, increased alertness and continual fear of threat can be advantageous in very short-lived conflict or challenging situations, it does become detrimental to our wellbeing in day-to-day living.

Should a state of hyper-arousal continue for weeks, months or even years, it will manifest in personality shifts that include emotional volatility and explosiveness, heightened aggression, agitation, skittishness, dissociative behaviour and insomnia. Reduced NPY concentrations in the brain are linked to PTSD.[32]

12 performance benefits associated with NPY:

- Enhanced resilience
- Greater courage
- Reduced anxiety
- Reduced stress
- Better sleep
- Reduced fear
- Lower risk of PTSD following trauma
- Extinction of fear-associated memories
- Improved concentration
- Reduced aggression and impulsivity
- Reduced alcohol cravings
- Improved mood.

Other ways to increase NPY expression include intermittent fasting or caloric restriction,[33] cold immersion[34] and certain adaptogens (a group of plants and herbs that have been shown to help our bodies respond to stress, anxiety, fatigue and promote a general state of overall balance). These include curcumin (a compound found in turmeric, a member of the ginger family) and Rhodiola rosea (a flowering plant that grows naturally in the wild Arctic regions of Europe, Asia and North America) and several others.[35]

The Mediterranean diet

The Mediterranean diet is arguably the best studied model of nutrition to date. This popular lifestyle is characterised by a high consumption of olive oil, vegetables, fruit, legumes, nuts, fish, low-fat dairy products, unrefined grains and a moderate intake of alcohol (principally red wine) and poultry. The consumption of red meat, processed or refined foods and sugars are kept to a minimum. Countless studies confirm an inverse relationship between the Mediterranean diet and inflammatory markers. One review article involving 17 studies showed 23,000 individuals over a period of 10 years who followed the Mediterranean diet were associated with a 23 per cent reduction in IL-6 below standard reference values.[36] The results experienced by being on the diet are commensurate with the degree of commitment shown to the long-established eating plan. This can in itself be motivating.

In a two-year Greek study involving 3,042 participants free of cardiovascular disease, those that were in the top third for Mediterranean diet compliance (i.e. the recommended daily consumption of fresh fruits, vegetables, olive oil, whole grains, fish) showed IL-6 and CRP levels that were 17 per cent and 20 per cent lower respectively than those in the bottom third.[37]

The Mediterranean diet can be adapted according to individual preference and lifestyle choices, provided the core principles are observed (i.e. lots of fruit and vegetables, fibre, olive oil, unrefined grains, wild fish, etc.).

The Mediterranean diet

Food type	Portions per day/week	Examples	Considerations
Unrefined grains and root vegetables	Daily	Brown and wild rice, oats, buckwheat, sweet potato, wholegrain bread and pasta	Some people may limit gluten-containing foods (wheat, barley, rye) due to underlying intolerances
Fruits	4–6 servings/day	Locally sourced	Seasonal and preferably organic
Vegetables	3 servings/day	Locally sourced	Seasonal and organic
Olive oil	With meals	Cold pressed, extra virgin	Used as a replacement for butter and animal fats
Low-fat dairy	1–2 portions/day	Yoghurt, unprocessed cheeses	Organic products where possible
Fish and poultry	3–4 portions/week	Sardines, salmon, hake/cod, tuna and other local fish	Preferably wild sourced and contamination free (i.e. from mercury and organochlorines), poultry should be free-range or ideally organic
Legumes, olives, potatoes	4–6 servings/week	Locally sourced	Organic products where possible
Nuts	4–6 portions/week	Walnuts, almonds, cashews, pecans, pistachios, Brazil nuts	Preferably raw, as opposed to flavoured, salted and roasted
Eggs	1–3 servings/week		Organic/free-range
Sweets and desserts	1–2 servings/week		Try to space it out, i.e. not having desserts in consecutive meals
Red meat and meat products	4 servings/month	Beef, lamb, venison, etc., including some processed meats	Free-range or organic
Wine	1–2 glasses/day		Choose organic or sulfite-free wine when available

Low-fat/low-carb diets

Unlike the Mediterranean diet or vegetarian eating plans, research into the low-fat or low-carb diets have produced very conflicting results in the regulation of inflammation and overall health promotion. Within the studies that do support improved immune regulation following either of these dietary approaches, it is almost always directly proportionate to how much weight participants lose during the trial period. In simple terms, if you are able to lose weight by being on a low-fat or low-carb diet, your immune system will respond favourably.

A scientifically formulated anti-inflammatory diet

In 2020 a passionate team of researchers and specialists from the Department of Medicine and Psychiatry at the University of California and the Department of Medicine at Autonomous University of Barcelona developed a dietary model known as the anti-inflammatory (ITIS) diet, a super-charged version of the Mediterranean diet.

The diet includes a few items that the traditional Mediterranean diet doesn't advocate, such as including a morning green drink, fermented foods, high-enzyme fruits, green tea, turmeric and ginger. At the same time, it requires the restriction of gluten, eggplant (aubergine), potatoes, tomatoes (nightshades) and the combining of grains and proteins at meals. It was aimed at addressing and supporting one of the most debilitating inflammatory diseases in existence – rheumatoid arthritis.[38] This autoimmune disorder causes excruciating and debilitating pain, swelling, stiffness, a loss of function in the joints and is associated with an extremely high (38.8 per cent) prevalence of depression and anxiety.[39] Raised IL-6 stands at the centre of this disease (and many other inflammatory disorders) acting through a variety of mechanisms.[40]

This means that for any diet plan to work, lowering, or at the very least stabilising, IL-6 is central to the strategy. The carry-over affect to resilience is that by reducing IL-6 one is able to reduce stress-related disorders, protect against depression and anxiety and reduce vulnerability to adversity.[41]

The ITIS diet

PLAN	RATIONALE	PRACTICAL APPLICATION
Fats and oils		
Increase daily intake of omega-3 fatty acids	Reduced inflammation	Twice weekly: sardines, tuna, salmon or other types of cold-water fish Daily consumption of: flax seeds, chia seeds, pumpkin seeds (based on tolerance)
Increase overall HEALTHY fat intake	Helps with the absorption of many nutrients and supports the immune, cardiovascular, hormonal and nervous systems	Daily consumption of: nuts (provided you don't have an allergy), avocado, sesame seeds, olive oil, unsalted raw nuts
Decrease intake of trans and saturated fats (found in animal products and processed foods)	Industrially produced trans fats and saturated fats have been shown to increase inflammation	Limit: pre-cooked foods, take-out, red meat, fried foods, high-fat dairy products
Gut health		
Increase daily intake of fibre	Improved overall immune regulation	Daily intake of: green leafy vegetables, fruits and hypoallergenic whole grains (sweet potato, brown rice, buckwheat, gluten-free oats) Avoid or limit: refined flours (incl. gluten-free)
Ensure daily intake of probiotics	Reduces expression of proinflammatory cytokines	Include: fermented foods (yoghurt, miso) or take high-quality probiotic supplement. Lactobacillus casei has been shown to be particularly beneficial

PLAN	RATIONALE	PRACTICAL APPLICATION
Digestion and dairy		
Support digestion of large proteins and prevent unnecessary fermentation, bloating and gas	Fibre helps protein digestion and reduces colonic transit The enzymes bromelain and papain have been shown to have an anti-inflammatory effect Large proteins in dairy (namely casein) are not completely digested and may feed harmful bacteria resulting in intestinal inflammation	Daily intake of: enzymatic fruits, such as pineapple, papaya, mango (which are all good sources of bromelain, papain and other proteolytic enzymes) Dissociate proteins from grains, i.e. eat proteins with vegetables Increase fibre intake Limit dairy: substitute milk with organic non-chemically treated plant-based milks (rice, oat, almond)
Herbs and spices		
Include more herbs and spices in food preparation	Turmeric, black pepper and ginger have antioxidant and anti-inflammatory properties	Include: turmeric, black pepper, ginger, sage, oregano, cinnamon, nutmeg, chilli, paprika and thyme
Limit salt	A high salt intake is associated with an increased risk of inflammatory diseases	Avoid or reduce: pre-cooked foods, salty snacks (salted and roasted nuts, chips, pretzels, biltong)
Vegetables		
Limit the consumption of vegetables from the nightshade family	They contain glycoalkaloids, which may increase intestinal permeability (allowing bacteria and undigested food materials to enter the body)	Avoid or limit: eggplant (aubergine), tomato (green), potato (especially the skin), all peppers
Increase overall vegetable intake	Vegetables with a high content of phytochemicals have been shown to have significant anti-inflammatory properties	Increase daily intake of: broccoli, cauliflower, garlic, onion, pumpkin, butternut, zucchini (courgette) and dark green leafy vegetables. Organic sources are preferable

PLAN	RATIONALE	PRACTICAL APPLICATION
Meat and proteins		
Decrease overall consumption of red meat	Red meat contains high levels of choline which is a precursor to the inflammatory molecule Trimethylamine N-oxide (TMAO)	Replace red meat with: legumes (lentils, chickpeas, beans), poultry and fish (2–3 times a week). It isn't uncommon to experience intolerances to some of the legumes so let your intuition be your guide.
Gluten and grains		
Reduce the overall consumption of some gluten-containing foods (wheat, barley, rye and spelt)	Gluten has been associated with inflammatory states	Daily: substitute refined wheat, barley and rye for corn, oats, quinoa, buckwheat, millet and brown rice
Processed and refined sugar		
Avoid refined sugars, all sugary foods and sugary beverages	Sugary foods are associated with obesity, changes to the bacterial colonies that reside in the digestive tract (the microbiome) and potentially a low-grade inflammatory state	Substitute with raw honey, seasonal fruit, dark chocolate, dates
Hot beverages		
Replace coffee with green and other herbal teas	The plant chemicals (polyphenols) found in green tea have been shown to decrease inflammation	Daily intake is suggested
Vitamins, antioxidants and plant-derived nutrients (phytochemicals)		
Increase intake of micronutrients and phytochemicals	Many antioxidant and phytochemicals have anti-inflammatory properties	Increase intake of vegetables, fruits, apple cider vinegar and whole grains (gluten-free)

Nutraceuticals

In recent years, the nutritional supplement (nutraceutical) industry (i.e. vitamins, minerals, botanicals, enzymes, amino acids and probiotics) has exploded, fuelled by a growing population who are desperately trying to gain control over their health and improve performance amid the volatility and uncertainty of our time.

In 2020 the research company MarketsandMarkets valued the world-wide nutraceutical industry at $136.2 billion annually.[42] In 2026 the sector is expected to be worth $204.7 billion. Despite a growing body of research supporting the value of targeted supplementation, there is still much scepticism (and I believe rightly so) within the industry, largely due to appalling regulations, tainted products, misguided application and the simple fact that a good proportion of nutraceuticals are simply ineffective in supporting their advertised benefits. There are, however, many compounds available that if sourced from a reputable supplier and taken correctly have the potential to promote resilience, reduce stress, improve health and reduce the risk of disease. Within the framework of resilience, there are some star performers, which include ashwagandha, resveratrol and quercetin and many herbal extracts that have the potential to greatly support resilience, overall health and performance.

THE ALL-STARS – ASHWAGANDHA, RESVERATROL AND QUERCETIN

There are many nutritional supplements that have proven effective in inhibiting IL-6 and thereby promoting resilience. One of the more potent IL-6 inhibitors is the adaptogen ashwagandha.

Ashwagandha is also known as Withania somnifera or Indian ginseng. It is a herb that has been used extensively in Ayurvedic medicine for thousands of years. This plant is from the nightshade family (other members of this plant family include tomatoes, potatoes and peppers) and is one of the most widely researched adaptogens. It has been studied in relation to its antioxidant, anti-carcinogenic, anti-anxiety, antidepressant, cardio-protective, thyroid-modulating, immune-modulating, anti-bacterial, anti-fungal, anti-inflammatory, neuroprotective and cognitive-enhancing effects. Over 35 chemical constituents have been isolated from ashwagandha, which have been shown to protect cells from oxidative damage and disease across a variety of research settings.

In 2021 a large team of Indian researchers performed a randomised placebo-controlled trial testing the efficacy of ashwagandha and other adaptogens in supporting recovery from COVID-19. A twice-daily oral dose of 500 mg of ashwagandha, along with three additional herbal compounds, was given for seven days to a treatment group of 45 individuals. In the placebo group, 50 patients received identical-looking tablets and drops. On day one and seven of the study, levels of the key inflammatory markers, IL-6, TNF-α and CRP, were meticulously measured. While the immune markers from both groups were comparable on day one, by day seven there was a large disparity. IL-6 levels in the treatment group were 250 per cent lower, as was CRP by 1,240 per cent and TNF-α by a staggering 2,000 per cent. Even more remarkable was that all of the patients in the treatment group made a full recovery (in only a week), compared to 60 per cent in the placebo group.[43]

Numerous studies done on ashwagandha have shown extraordinary outcomes within a wide dosage range and application, and aside from reductions in the major inflammatory markers, especially IL-6, the stress hormones epinephrine and cortisol, blood glucose and lipids also show marked decreases.[44][45]

Serotonin and GABA

Yet another powerful benefit attributed to an ongoing (three weeks or longer) ashwagandha supplementation is its positive affect on serotonin and GABA, neurochemicals known for their role in resilience and human potential.[46] We know that serotonin influences mood, sleep and emotional behaviours, but what is less well known is the role this molecule plays in the promotion of human connection, learning, memory, cognitive flexibility and, most notably, the modulation of immune behaviours.[47]

GABA is the mind's natural calming signal. Its role is to promote relaxation, a sense of tranquility, improved sleep and relieve stress and anxiety. It also acts to balance the effects of glutamate, the stimulatory neurochemical that is dramatically elevated as a result of neuroinflammation.

Risks and considerations

Before taking any nutritional supplement, especially an adaptogen, it is important to speak to your physician or healthcare practitioner. This is especially important if you have an underlying health condition or family history of health compromise.

The current body of literature reports a low level of toxicity in ashwagandha, even at extremely high doses. However, it is vital to exercise caution when combining ashwagandha with any medication, especially first-generation antidepressants, specifically monoamine oxidase inhibitors (MAOIs). Many nutrients and medications have been shown to have negative interactions with MAOIs, which is why this class of medication has, in many cases, been replaced with newer generation options.

Current dosage guidelines for ashwagandha

Lowest effective dose	50–100 mg/day
Suggested dose	300–500 mg/day
Higher dose ranges (still within safety limits)	1,000–6,000 mg/day

Finally, if you are pregnant, nursing or suffer with a nightshade allergy (tomatoes, potatoes, eggplant (aubergine), peppers, etc.), it will be wise to steer clear of the adaptogen, as ashwagandha belongs to the same family.

For maximum effectiveness

Ashwagandha root extract is the preferred form for the purposes of supplementation and is best taken with meals, ideally with breakfast.

Resveratrol and quercetin

Other adaptogens, such as resveratrol and quercetin, have been shown to have astounding resilience benefits and have both been personal favourites of mine for many years. Resveratrol is a polyphenol that is found in over 70 plant species, including blueberries, grapes, cacao and peanuts and has been linked to many life extension advantages. So much so that it is strongly endorsed by Dr David Sinclair, a professor of genetics at Harvard Medical School, who is the world authority in the ageing space. Over and above resveratrol's potent immune-modulating properties, this plant compound has powerful neuroprotective and mood-supporting effects.

A word of caution

Very high doses of resveratrol (exceeding 2.5 grams per day) may be associated with some side effects, which include nausea, vomiting, diarrhoea and potentially liver dysfunction. Another issue with extreme doses is the potential for increased cell damage and stress;[48] an opposite response can be seen with lower to moderate intakes.

Quercetin, known for its positive influence on oxytocin, is widely regarded as a long-lasting anti-inflammatory substance with tremendous immune-modulatory capacities.[49] Like many of the adaptogens, quercetin offers many health benefits beyond its influence on the immune system, such as

Current dosage guidelines for resveratrol and quercetin and the profound influence on the proinflammatory cytokines

Nutrient	Influence on IL-6 expression	Influence on TNF-α expression	Suggested daily dose
Resveratrol	↓ 100%	↓ 79%	150–445 mg
Quercetin	↓ 98%	↓ 43%	1–2 g

fighting free radicals and protecting against neurological diseases. While there are no obvious side effects from quercetin supplementation, it is important to be mindful that it may interact with some medications.[50] If you are on any medication, speak to your doctor first.

Herbs and spices

Decades of research in the field of nutrition has shown that a diet high in fruits, vegetables, herbs and spices promotes health, vitality and offers significant protection against many inflammatory diseases.[51][52] A 2010 study published in the journal *Food Chemistry* screened a range of foods and compounds for their anti-inflammatory activity, using the standard model for studying and evaluating pharmaceuticals (lipopolysaccharide [LPS] stimulated macrophages).[53] The study revealed that several plant extracts and compounds not only inhibit IL-6 and other proinflammatory molecules, such as TNF-α, but they also have the potential to elevate the potent anti-inflammatory protein known as interleukin 10 (IL-10). This increase in IL-10 expression can constrain many of the primary inflammatory pathways as well as the microglia, the brain's intrinsic immune system, which has the potential to translate into improved health and significant resilience. Some of the most potent anti-inflammatory foods might surprise you, as they include chilli, black pepper, sage, oregano, cinnamon and nutmeg.

These numbers further support the fact that a balanced plant-rich diet can be powerful in the promotion of resilience and reduce vulnerability

Top 10 herbs and spices in reducing inflammation

Food/spice	Influence on IL-6 expression
Chilli	↓ 81%
Black pepper	↓ 90%
Cinnamon	↓ 57%
Ginger	↓ 50%
Ginseng	↓ 12%
Nutmeg	↓ 70%
Oregano	↓ 49%
Paprika	↓ 28%
Sage	↓ 62%
Thyme	↓ 26%

to adversity. The key to creating a successful outcome is to find small opportunities throughout the day to incorporate these foods. For example, add cinnamon (generously) to your morning oats or muesli. Crush black pepper on your savoury snacks throughout the course of the day. Add paprika, sage, oregano and chilli (if you enjoy it) liberally to your food while you're cooking.

PLANT EXTRACTS HOLD THEIR OWN AGAINST CORTISONE

Cortisone, the synthetic form of cortisol, is widely used in managing inflammatory diseases and health issues related to immune dysregulation. Very few medications are effective in this regard as anyone who has used cortisone for any length of time can testify.

The study published in *Food Chemistry* compared the effects of cortisol (which is produced by the body as opposed to cortisone, which is a synthetic derivative) to many of the anti-inflammatory extracts found in vegetables and fruits, herbs and spices. While cortisol did lower IL-6 and TNF-α, it was overshadowed in its potential by at least nine plant extracts, including apigenin (found in chamomile, sage, thyme, parsley), capsaicin (found in chilli peppers), quercetin (found in apples, berries, parsley), luteolin (found in rosemary, sage, thyme, parsley) and resveratrol (found in red wine, grapes, pistachios, blueberries and cacao).

Where cortisol does have an extra advantage is its ability to regulate inflammatory pathways (as opposed to dampening proinflammatory responses), as measured by the increased expression of IL-10 to the extent of 130 per cent.

The simple message is that by simply adding more herbs and spices to our foods, we can better support our health and create a better platform for improved resilience.

This section has highlighted the power of health behaviours in shaping our reality, both in the present and in the future. By choosing to exercise more frequently and being more deliberate in the type of exercise and the intensity and timing of our activity, we pave the way for extraordinary performance, driven largely by immune modulation and greater neurochemical expression and balance. At the same time, the foods and supplements we choose for ourselves further contribute to the realisation of our dreams, aspirations and ability to navigate this complex world, which is filled with endless and unrelenting challenges.

■

SECTION SUMMARY

- The negative behaviours and activities that lower resilience include excessive alcohol intake, sleep deprivation, high intakes of processed sugar, smoking and chronic psychological stress.
- Exercise and a healthy diet promote resilience through improved immune regulation.
- Exercise increases and supports BDNF, serotonin and dopamine.
- Physical activity is associated with lowered inflammation due to an increase in more than eight anti-inflammatory factors, including IL-10 and BDNF.
- While all forms of physical exercise lower inflammation, high-intensity interval training (HIIT) offers the greatest benefit. This is largely due to higher reductions in body fat, greater elevations in BDNF (when compared to moderate-intensity protocols), increased growth hormone release and enhanced mental toughness through developing a physical tolerance to pain.
- A 10–30 per cent increase in BDNF expression and signalling enhances cognition, creativity, memory and IQ. It also protects against depression and anxiety.
- Any diet plan that is able to achieve and maintain optimal weight will promote resilience.
- Vegan or plant-based diets are associated with a 72 per cent lower systemic inflammation when compared to mixed diets.
- The primary benefit of plant-based diets within the context of immune regulation and improved resilience is a high fibre content.
- Lower animal protein consumption is associated with raised levels of NPY, a molecule with exceptional resilience-promoting effects.
- The Mediterranean diet is the most studied of all dietary models. It is characterised by a high consumption of olive oil, fresh vegetables, seasonal and local fruits, legumes, nuts, fish and unrefined grains,

with moderate intakes of wine, poultry and low-fat dairy. Refined carbohydrates and sugars, processed foods and red meat are kept to a minimum.

- Long-term adherence to the Mediterranean diet is associated with a 23 per cent reduction in inflammatory markers below standard reference values.
- Many nutrients have been shown to reduce inflammation and improve resilience. The star performers in this regard are ashwagandha, quercetin and resveratrol.
- Several common herbs and spices have been shown to have exceptional anti-inflammatory properties. Some of the more potent foods and compounds include chilli, black pepper, cinnamon, ginger, nutmeg, oregano, paprika, sage and thyme.

WHAT IS YOUR PERSONAL RESILIENCE SCORE?

THE REFLECTION TEST

This foundational resilience assessment will help you to objectively see where your strengths and weaknesses lie. It is based on the seven major areas, which means that if you score low (under 50 per cent) for a particular area, you can refer to the relevant section in the book for action steps. The assessment is for a maximum score of 102 points.

Scoring

Very resilient: 90–102 points
Resilient: 70–89 points
Moderate resilience: 50–69 points
Not yet resilient: 0–49 points

Personality	Yes, definitely (3 points)	Sometimes (2 points)	Seldom (1 point)	Never (0 points)
I am outgoing and even extroverted at times				
I am optimistic				
I am conscientious				
I am open to new experiences				
I am agreeable (forgiving, empathetic, modest)				
I am generally considered to be a calm person				
SECTION SCORE				**/18 points**

Current environment	Yes, definitely (3 points)	Sometimes (2 points)	Seldom (1 point)	Never (0 points)
My home and/or work environment is a positive and encouraging one				
I would describe my close relationships as attentive and caring				
I am surrounded by support, compassion and concern				
SECTION SCORE				/9 points

Refining existing coping mechanisms and developing new ones	Yes, definitely (3 points)	Sometimes (2 points)	Seldom (1 point)	Never (0 points)
I am constantly striving to improve my existing skills and abilities				
I am committed to learning new skills, even though the process itself can be difficult and at times frustrating				
SECTION SCORE				/6 points

My early years	Never (3 points)	Seldom (2 points)	Sometimes (1 point)	Sadly, yes (0 points)
I grew up with uncertainty and volatility (socio-economic)				
I felt neglected, uncared for or unloved at times				
I was subjected to emotional abuse				
I was subjected to physical or sexual abuse and/or trauma (major injury, surgery, disease)				
SECTION SCORE				/12 points

Cognitive reappraisal	Yes, definitely (3 points)	Sometimes (2 points)	Seldom (I point)	Never (0 points)
I see setbacks, failures and challenges as an opportunity to improve myself and grow				
I am able to find meaning in many of the challenges you experience				
I sometimes find myself reinterpreting the details of stressful events to make them appear less negative				
SECTION SCORE				**/9 points**
Mastery over stress responses	Yes, definitely (3 points)	Sometimes (2 points)	Seldom (I point)	Never (0 points)
I have special people in my life (parents, friends, partner) that make me feel safe and protected				
I have good emotional support structures				
I am able to manage my stress (through exercise, therapies, nutritional supplements, diet)				
I practise mindfulness or other forms of meditation regularly				
SECTION SCORE				**/12 points**
Immunity	Yes, definitely (3 points)	Sometimes (2 points)	Seldom (I point)	Never (0 points)
Do you believe you can achieve most things you set your mind to?				
Do you set yourself short- and longer-term goals?				

Immunity (*continued*)	Yes, definitely (3 points)	Sometimes (2 points)	Seldom (1 point)	Never (0 points)
Do you engage in activities that bring you joy and happiness?				
Do you have people in your life that make you laugh and smile daily?				
Do you believe that your future holds great promise?				
Do you believe you have the ability to influence the direction of your life?				
Do you perform aerobic exercise at least three times a week?				
Do you exercise vigorously at least once a week (e.g. CrossFit, HIIT, competitive sport)?				
Is your weight within normal range (i.e. BMI 18.5–24.9)?				
Do you follow a diet that is high in fibre and that limits red meat, refined carbohydrates, processed sugar and dairy?				
Are you taking two or more of the following supplements: omega-3 fatty acids, vitamin D, probiotics, quercetin, ashwagandha, resveratrol, curcumin?				
Do you include herbs and spices in food preparation, i.e. black pepper, oregano, cinnamon, sage, paprika, thyme, etc?				
SECTION SCORE				/36 points
			TOTAL SCORE	/102 points

Putting it all together

Personality matters
Resilience is supported by being more outgoing, conscientious, optimistic, agreeable and open.
Practical application: focus on building one or two of these character traits.

Create the right environment for yourself
Build a space that is positive, encouraging, attentive, caring, compassionate, empathetic and supportive.

Consider gene testing for you and/or your family and/or team
The gene panel selection should include HTTLPR, COMT, DRD4, FKBP5, BDNF, OXTR and MAOA.

Exposure to childhood adversity requires a long-term stress management commitment
Being exposed to abuse, neglect or uncertainty in our formative years demands that we create a long-term plan for stress management.

Refine and improve your existing resilience skills
Practical application: write a list of your current strengths and vulnerabilities together with action steps that will support improvement.

Strive to grow and build on to your existing resilience set
Focus areas should include the practice of cognitive reappraisal, strengthening support systems, habit formation and motivation, developing confidence and a strong leaning to health promotion.

The best time to develop resilience is early in life due to the plasticity of the brain during these periods.

Resilience has a defined neural signature that includes increased brain volume and recruitment in those areas that support attention and focus, decision-making, planning, impulse control and memory. Additionally, resilience is supported by reduced connectivity between the amygdala and the major brain networks.

Turning back the clock
Positive changes in brain structure can be achieved through meditation practice and ongoing supplementation with omega-3 fatty acids.

Intellect and emotional regulation govern resilience. One of the more effective resilience skills is cognitive reappraisal.

There are three primary cognitive reappraisal strategies. They are psychological distancing, challenging reality and changing circumstances. A good way to measure cognitive reappraisal is through psycholinguistics.

Cognitive reappraisal is highly dependent on raised levels and activity of catecholamines (dopamine, norepinephrine and ephinephrine). Therefore COMT enzyme expression is a strong determinant of reframing potential. To reduce COMT enzyme expression, which will increase dopamine, perform aerobic exercise on a regular basis and/or supplement with Bacopa monnieri.

Master your stress responses
While many stress management strategies exist, social support and buffering offer unparalled benefits. These include reduced activity in the brain's fear centres, increased activity in the executive regions, together with increased expression of oxytocin.

Mindfulness-based stress reduction combats the effects of loneliness and supports stress modulation.
Oxytocin supports resilience and protects against the negative influence of a lack of social connection. Oxytocin expression can be increased with exercise, yoga or supplementation of quercetin, vitamin D, Lactobacillus reuteri, vitamin C and magnesium.

Resilience is largely governed by immune behaviours
Neuroinflammation reduces serotonin, dopamine and BDNF. It also increases glutamate and stress responses.

The resilience biomarker IL-6 can be better regulated by exercising personal control, being more positive and being optimistic.

Health behaviours support immune regulation and improve resilience
Try to exercise regularly (intensely from time to time, health permitting), reduce red meat, processed sugar, refined carbohydrate, fried foods, excessive dairy and possibly even gluten. At the same time, increase your intake of fermented foods, fibre, fresh vegetables and seasonal fruits, unrefined grains, omega-3 fatty acids, with cold water fish and digestive enzymes. Herbs and spices, as well as ashwagandha, resveratrol and quercetin, also have an incredibly powerful effect on immune regulation and overall health.

PART 3

LESSONS IN RESILIENCE FROM OLYMPIC CHAMPIONS – A MASTERCLASS IN BEHAVIOURAL SCIENCE

STRESS IS BEHIND
EVERY SUCCESS

Since I was a young boy, I was captivated by exceptional sporting performance and the energy, excitement and mystery of it. I'd constantly wonder how it was possible that elite athletes could achieve such high levels of skill and accomplishment. To me, it was nothing short of superhuman.

Watching my childhood heroes, including Martina Navratilova and Ivan Lendl, helped me momentarily transcend the challenges and struggles in my life and helped me believe that anything was possible if you worked hard enough. These sporting stars were the embodiment of this.

Unfortunately, like so many children, I was not in an environment that supported or encouraged my personal and sporting development. But the lure of sport and the sporting world was always strong within me.

When adults asked what I wanted to be when I grew up, I always responded that I wanted to work with the world's best athletes and help them become faster, stronger, fitter and healthier. Essentially, I wanted to help them succeed. There was never any doubt in my mind that this was what I wanted to do.

But it was the early 1980s and my choice of a so-called "career" was somewhat frowned upon. "That is not a career" usually followed my enthusiastic response. "What about becoming a doctor, an accountant or even a restaurateur?" While these other options were appealing, I stuck to my guns and this often elicited sighing, head shaking and eye rolling from the adults. "How exactly are you going to achieve this?" some would ask. Probing a 12-year-old for a 20-year business strategy always ended the conversation. As a child, I had no idea how I was going to do it, but I knew that my *only* strengths were passion, drive and bundles of hope.

Fast-forward 20 years and I was working with some of the world's most iconic athletes (including my childhood icon – Martina Navratilova) and teams. When first entering the world of professional sport, I was astounded by the hardships and challenges that athletes faced on a daily basis. The life of a professional athlete that we see on social media, in the media and on billboards in no way reflects their gruelling and harsh reality.

To help understand this world better a comprehensive analysis of 34 studies, involving 1,809 individuals, showed that athletes experience approximately 640 distinct stressors on an ongoing basis.[1] These stressors can be divided into 29 subcategories, which fall into four main categories

Common stressors experienced by professional athletes

Leadership & public	Team & culture	Environment	Performance & personal issues
• Coaches' behaviours and interactions • Coaches' personality and attitudes • Expectations • Support staff • Officials and governing body • Media and spectators	• Teammates – behaviour and interaction • Communication • Atmosphere and support • Norms and roles • Goals	• Facilities and equipment • Selection process • Training • Travel • Regulations • Distractions • Safety • Technology • No distinction between work and non-work activities	• Injuries • Illness • Finances • Diet and lifestyle expectations • Career transitions • Relationships • Loneliness • Fatigue • Failures and performance slumps

that include issues surrounding leadership and personnel, team and team culture, and environment and personal challenges.

Prior to COVID-19, many of these stressors would have been foreign to most of us and completely unrelatable. But in the new reality we all find ourselves in, it is striking how everyday stresses echo those historically and currently found in the world of professional sport. Fragmented relationships, loneliness, isolation, disappointments, repeated failures, work–family conflict, fatigue, illness, physical pain, careers that end abruptly, extended work days and weeks, all compounded with ongoing financial pressure are now collective experiences that we can all relate to.

However, the major distinction is that we didn't choose this reality, nor did we sign up for the plethora of additional stresses that now overwhelm our lives due to the changes that have occurred over the last few years. Unlike us, athletes choose this life and, at the highest level, actively seek to engage with challenging and difficult situations, day in, day out.

Interestingly, almost all theories of resilience are based on clinical populations (children, adults, families, communities) who, through no choice of their own, have been forced to react to traumatic and stressful events in their lives. Resilience in these populations is therefore a prerequisite for coping and the maintenance of basic functioning.

This is what makes the current body of research into athletes and resilience so relatable and applicable to our own lives. The findings are relevant to high achievers in all areas of life who actively place themselves in demanding situations to raise their performance level and overall success prospects. The learnings offer us the tools for an improved capacity to handle pressure and adversity and to realise our fullest potential in both favourable and adverse conditions.

Over the last few decades there has been a substantial volume of research into understanding resilience from an athletic and sporting perspective. During this time the study that has been most impactful (certainly in my work with high-performing teams and individuals) has been *A Grounded*

Theory of Psychological Resilience in Olympic Champions by David Fletcher from Loughborough University and Mustafa Sarkar from Nottingham Trent University.[2]

This groundbreaking study, published back in 2012, sought to explore and elucidate the relationship between psychological resilience and elite sport performance. Many studies done over the years have shown that Olympic gold medallists have psychological traits that set them apart from less accomplished athletes. With this understanding, 12 Olympic champions (both male and female) representing a range of sports (both individual and team), from four different countries, were interviewed regarding their experiences of adversity, setbacks, pressures, failures and successes during their long and eventful sporting careers.

The findings revealed that Olympic champions have an arsenal of powerful psychological factors and core behaviours that protect them from the potential negative effects of stress and adversity. These psychological traits offer protection against vulnerability under some of the most extreme conditions and also ensure success at times when it matters the most, such as when there is pressure to perform and deliver exceptional results.

None of the athletes in the study were exempt or free of ongoing adversity and challenge throughout their careers. In fact, every member of the group encountered significant hardships on an ongoing basis, and the only difference between them was the frequency, intensity and duration of adversity.

The study found that Olympic champions experience stress from three distinct sources:

1. Competitive stresses (formidable opponents, loss of form, increased self-doubt, poor performances).
2. Organisational issues (politics, unwavering demands, administrative hurdles).

3. Personal challenges (sport–family conflict, injuries, poor health, fatigue).

As challenging as this collective set may be, what the study and its rigorous interview process revealed was that it was the stress and adversity itself that led to Olympic success.

According to Fletcher and Sarkar: "It is important to emphasise that exposure to stressors was an essential feature of the stress–resilience–performance relationship in Olympic champions. Indeed, most of the participants argued that if they had not experienced certain types of stressors at specific times, including highly demanding adversities such as parental divorce, serious illness and career-threatening injuries, they would not have won their gold medals."

Some of the most powerful resilience skills that exist within this group of champions include cognitive reappraisal, metacognition and positive personality. There are practical ways we can develop and grow these skills and incorporate them into our own lives.

CHAMPION SKILL #1

COGNITIVE REAPPRAISAL

I really think a champion is defined not by their wins but by how they can recover when they fall.

SERENA WILLIAMS

Of the many resilience- and performance-promoting psychological strategies in the Olympic champion repertoire, cognitive reappraisal is the core behaviour that most effectively supports success in adversity.

Reframing had become such a fundamental part of who the Olympians were and what they represented that they genuinely perceived stressors, setbacks, failures, disappointments, obstacles and frustrations as opportunities for personal growth, athletic development and self-mastery. In addition, the closer they were to their athletic potential (i.e. the better form they were in) at the time of the challenge or stress experience, the more they were able to see the opportunity that was embedded within the crisis itself. Overcoming hardships and hurdles appears to fuel Olympic champions in the sense that they perceive a psychological and competitive edge over their opposition.

For many of us, a significant event or personal failure during the peak of our careers can profoundly affect our confidence, self-belief and even our desire to continue in our chosen endeavours. It shakes us to the core, and finding opportunity, let alone meaning, in those situations is near impossible as we fixate our attention on the external factors that contributed to the derailment. Yet, if we pause briefly, have the courage to remove ego from the situation and reflect with objectivity, there is often a gift implanted within the entire experience.

During the more than two decades I spent immersed in professional sport, I can recall countless examples of elite athletes overcoming major setbacks and disappointments through a cognitive reappraisal. That said, one of the greatest examples of this core resilience skill is unquestionably the British track and field champion Jonathan Edwards.

When Jonathan was a boy, he had a passion for sport and was good at just about every sport he participated in, receiving numerous awards for sporting excellence. However, believing the opinions of the adults around him that professional sport was not a career option, he always kept a strong work ethic and a commitment to his academic studies and was a recipient of his school's top award for academic excellence.

His passion was the triple jump and although he had won the English Schools Championship title at the age of 18 in 1984, by international standards and the traditional matrix of performance and development, Edwards was way off the pace – his distances were not overly special. Yet, his father believed in him and his abilities and pushed him to keep working on his triple jump throughout his school career.

Jonathan went to Durham University to study physics and, at the age of 21, the athletics bug was as strong as ever. He decided that once he had completed his degree, he would concentrate his efforts on full-time professional sport. His greatest attribute was his speed, which in the triple jump is foundational – there was hope he could develop his sporting career. Incredibly, within a short period following his decision to become a full-time athlete, Edwards qualified for the 1988 Olympics in Seoul, Korea. Although it was a dream come true for him, he was petrified and recalls: "Getting my kit, being in the same team as Daley Thompson, seeing Carl Lewis at the training camp. I remember thinking, what am I doing here?"

Of the 43 competitors, Edwards, a relative newcomer to full-time sport, placed 23rd, with a jump of 15.88 metres, only 2 metres shy of that year's gold medallist.

Edwards was off to an incredible start and the result motivated him to put his head down, train even harder, intensify his commitment to the sport and continue to grow and evolve as a triple jumper. If he was able to place 23rd in his first Olympics, the possibilities of what he could achieve four years later in the next Olympics were limitless. The four years passed and once again Edwards found himself competing at the Olympics in Barcelona, Spain. Would the five years as a full-time athlete (as opposed to only one year in the previous Olympics) be the differentiator from a results standpoint at this Olympics? He was, by his own admission, in the shape of his life!

Sadly, the Olympics turned out to be a major disappointment for Edwards. Despite his best efforts and the additional years of training, he placed 35th, with a jump of only 15.76 metres. He had actually gone backwards. Placed in the same situation, many of us would feel utterly despondent and demotivated. Five years of full-time sacrifice, constantly pushing his body to extremes, limited social interaction, strict dietary protocols, the daily monotony, injuries and pain and not only was he not moving forward, he was slowly regressing. For most people, with a good education as a fail-safe, this type of setback would be a formula for a career transition.

But Jonathan Edwards was not just anyone and his career was far from over. Using the failure to fuel himself, he was able to find the courage to push forward with even greater resolve than before.

In spite of his determined efforts and a bronze medal at the World Championships in 1993, the following two years' results were deeply disappointing. In 1994 Edwards experienced a further setback. After almost seven years as a full-time athlete, he contracted the Epstein-Barr virus. This virus is often associated with infectious mononucleosis, which has put the brakes on many athletic careers and even prematurely ended some. In the sport of tennis, stars like Roger Federer, Andy Murray, Andy Roddick and countless others have had to forgo at least an entire season in order to recover from this virus. There have been cases where athletes have never recovered and have had to retire.

Epstein-Barr is associated with chronic fatigue, weakness, fever and can lead to anaemia and inflammation of the heart, known as myocarditis. Symptoms typically last a month, but many sufferers can feel unwell for more than six months and experience relapses when overtraining or under chronic stress. This is precisely why athletes struggle with this particular virus.

If the sheer disappointment and failure at the Olympics in Barcelona hadn't shaken Jonathan's athletic dream enough, then being bedridden for weeks, or potentially months, would surely bring closure to a disappointing and challenging career. However, being the master reframer that he was, Edwards not only viewed the downtime as an opportunity for some much-needed rest and recovery, he also put his physics degree to good use. A deep understanding and application of the physics of motion can dramatically influence the speed, height and distance in any athletic endeavour, especially triple jumping. While in bed recovering from the virus, Edwards reflected deeply on his jumping technique and training and developed novel ways to further refine his training and development programme. He watched countless hours of video footage of himself and his rivals in terms of his technique analysis.

As a result, Edwards started the new year with a vastly improved jumping technique and was rested, with renewed drive and passion. In his first big event of 1995, Edwards broke the UK national record. Could the last eight years of hard work finally be paying off?

In June of that year, Jonathan was competing in the European Cup in Lille, France. In the warm-up, he was looking particularly explosive and feeling good. In his first round attempt, he jumped an incredible 17.90 metres. Considering that the world record at the time was 17.97 metres, this was a sensational result. He was elated and bursting with self-belief and confidence.He prepared himself for his second attempt. He raised his arms in the air to engage and mobilise the crowd, said a few words to himself, took a deep breath and launched into his sprint. According to triple-jump analysts at the time, every step, foot contact, motion and action was utterly flawless. He ended up jumping a staggering 18.43 metres – the longest jump ever recorded in the sport! Unfortunately, the wind speed that day was just over the legal threshold of 2.0 metres per second (it was 2.4 metres per seconds) and, as a result, the jump could not be considered a record. But it was clear that his time had come. Not only was he living up to his potential, he had redefined the parameters of the sport.

Several weeks later, Edwards officially broke the world record at a provincial meet in Spain, with a jump of 17.98 metres.

His form continued to improve throughout the 1995 summer season. The World Championships were held in August that year, the biggest and most important event of the year. As the current world record holder and "man to beat", going into the event was terrifying and pressurised. For the first time in Edwards' career, the expectations on him were high and it was a very different type of stress experience to what he was used to.

"Although I'd broken the world record that year already, in my mind had I not won the World Championships, my season would have been regarded as a failure," he said. "So I felt a huge amount of pressure because I'd never gone into a major championships expected to win. And not just expected to win but to break a world record as well, so I was petrified," said Edwards.

As anticipated, he flew into the final but was well aware that he was in the company of some of the biggest jumpers the sport had even known.

With all eyes on him, Edwards prepared for his first jump and exploded into a sprint, flew down the runway and took off, landing well beyond the 18-metre mark. He leapt into the air, arms raised, ecstatic. Within a few moments, it was official – Jonathan Edwards had broken his previous world record (that only stood for 20 days) with a jump of 18.16 metres! The 18-metre barrier had officially been broken.

"It was a celebration but also a huge amount of relief," recalled Edwards. But Jonathan wasn't done.

It was as if all of his past failures, struggles, setbacks, challenges, disappointments, hurdles and frustrations over the previous eight or more years seemed to connect as part of a large and complex plan to take him to the point of athletics perfection. Twenty minutes later, he was on the runway for round two, but the difference this time was that he had a smile on his face as he prepared for take-off. His routine remained the same and he said a few words to himself before exploding in the run. Again, he landed beyond the 18-metre mark. He was in disbelief, the crowd erupted and his competitors gasped. The official distance was 18.29 metres – he broke his previous world record, which had only been set a minute before. Jonathan Edwards is the only track and field athlete in history to set two world records in two consecutive attempts. Remarkably, his record still stands to this day.

Jonathan Edwards went on to win six European cups, the European Championships, two World Championships, the Commonwealth Games and the most prized victory in sport – an Olympic gold in Sydney in 2000.

THE GROWTH MINDSET

What Olympic champions ultimately showcase is what Stanford professor Carol S Dweck refers to as a "growth mindset'. In her must-read book, *Mindset: Changing the Way You Think to Fulfil Your Potential*, Dweck offers a simple premise: the world is divided into those who are open to learning (growth mindset) and those who are closed to it (closed mindset), and this trait ultimately impacts your potential throughout life.[1] A growth mindset is the belief that you can constantly cultivate and improve on your abilities through practice and effort, regardless of your circumstances.

By contrast, a fixed mindset is the belief that your abilities are predetermined and largely unchangeable. Having a fixed mindset will create a higher degree of vulnerability in the face of challenge and adversity, and this stems from the fact that failure of any kind is perceived as a personal reflection of someone's limited abilities and deeper fragility. Of course, these are nothing more than self-determined and imposed constructs that reflect the mindset itself. What is fascinating is that when deconstructed, the fear that is the driving force is being perceived by others as a disappointment. This results in a relentless drive to prove ourselves to the world over and over again.

For example, an athlete with a fixed mindset who is going through a performance slump would typically voice their frustrations in the following ways: Maybe this game isn't for me after all. Perhaps I'm not meant to be competing at this level of the sport. I try so hard, but nothing I do makes any difference. My team is useless – they are the issue!

In stark contrast, those Olympic athletes with a growth mindset don't let their failures define them. Instead, they perceive their failures as an opportunity to improve and move forward, just like Jonathan Edwards did. Armed with a growth mindset, Olympic champions and elite athletes in all sports see challenges as a vehicle that forces them to confront and address their current weaknesses and/or limitations, making them stronger in the process.

Their response to adversity is: This setback could be a good thing in the long run. I need to go back to the drawing board with my team. I am disappointed by the situation but I see where I need to improve. This failure hurts, but I can overcome it like everything else.

There are countless stories of great athletes, including soccer star Lionel Messi, the boxer Muhammad Ali and basketball player Michael Jordan, who were rejected, overlooked or sidelined in their youth because they weren't "good enough", "quick enough", "strong enough", "competitive enough" or unbelievably "tall enough'. Yet, they all turned their challenges and disappointments into growth opportunities and were able to convert their failures into hard work, greater skills development and an even stronger motivation to succeed.

What is your current mindset? Take this quick quiz to give you a measurable indicator.

The quiz is for a maximum score of 18 points.

Desired response	Yes, definitely (3 points)	Sometimes (2 points)	Seldom (1 point)
I see challenge as a growth opportunity			
I can learn and do almost anything I set my mind to			
I realise that success is largely determined by my efforts and attitude			
I am grateful for feedback from others, even if it's not always what I want to hear			
I find the success of others very inspiring			
I am open to trying new things, even if it means failing from time to time			

Scoring

Extremely growth orientated: 12–18 points

Good: 6–12 points

I have some work to do: 0–6 points

■

SECTION SUMMARY

- Professional athletes are confronted with countless stresses and obstacles on a daily basis. Their typical challenges include leadership and public demands, team dynamics and team culture, training and competitive environment, and personal issues.
- Athletes differ from other groups of people, in that they have chosen challenge and adversity as a way of life.
- Olympic champions and other highly accomplished athletes have developed a repertoire of effective behavioural and psychological strategies to help them navigate competitive and organisational stresses as well as ongoing personal challenges.
- Olympic champions view stress, failure, setbacks and adversity as an opportunity for personal growth, self-development and professional mastery.
- Olympic champions embody the "growth mindset", which is the belief that one can constantly cultivate and improve on one's abilities through practice and effort.
- Olympic champions don't allow their failures to define them.

CHAMPION SKILL #2

METACOGNITION

You can't put a limit on anything.
The more you dream, the farther you get.
MICHAEL PHELPS

In addition to seeing challenge and adversity, setbacks and failures, pain and hardship as opportunities to achieve greater levels of personal mastery, Olympic gold medallists are able to withstand the demands and pressure of high-level competition through a cognitive process known as metacognition. Metacognition is the ability to understand and control your thoughts and is dependent on greater self-awareness and self-mastery.

Metacognition allows us to recognise that we can't control many of the external circumstances and events that are continuously taking place around us, but we can control how we think. How we think then translates to how we feel. How we think and feel will determine what we say and how we use language. How we communicate effects our behaviours and, as we know, it is our behaviours and habits that create our reality in the long run.

Metacognition is a skill that can be developed through many behaviours, which include self-dialogue, goal setting, the use of imagery and even the conscious and deliberate manipulation of levels of arousal. The following section explores the characteristics that drive self-awareness and self-control and the ways we can apply them to our own lives and in our own context.

SELF-DIALOGUE

One of the most exciting tennis matches in recent years was the 2019 Wimbledon final between the maestro, Roger Federer, and the formidable Novak Djokovic. Both players had been perched at the top of world tennis for over a decade in what is considered to be one of the most competitive eras in men's tennis. Their head-to-head stats suggested a titanic battle, with Federer winning 22 of their encounters and Djokovic 25. Federer's advantage going into the match was eight previous Wimbledon titles compared to Djokovic's four. As expected, the match was tight, with both players doing their utmost to minimise unforced errors. However, Roger appeared to have an ascendancy, especially after taking the fourth set by breaking Novak's serve twice. The crowd, firmly behind Roger, erupted.

Just as the energy was reaching a fever pitch resembling that of a soccer match, not a Wimbledon final, Novak took a "comfort" break. A "comfort" break is something Djokovic takes frequently during tight matches. He uses it to re-centre himself and, in the context of turning the match around, he has an 83.3 per cent success rate following a trip to the men's locker room. During this strategic break at the end of the fourth set, in a post-match interview Novak described a conversation he had had with himself where he repeatedly told himself to be present, to be in the moment and to believe in his abilities. He encouraged others to use this technique too.

When Novak returned to the court, as the historical stats show, he was firmly back in the match. The fifth set lasted a staggering two hours and two minutes, with Djokovic saving two match points to beat Federer in one of the toughest encounters in tennis history.

So often our personal narrative during the difficult periods in our lives is despondent, negative and extremely self-critical. We tend to focus all our energy and attention on the overwhelming nature of the immediate challenge, the potential impossibility of the situation, what's not working, why it's not working, where we are failing, our shortcomings, our limitations and our inability to foresee the event unfolding, imagining no possible end or solution in sight. Yet, if we don't compound the external pressures with an internal struggle (i.e. self-condemnation and a sense of hopelessness), we choose to acknowledge the situation for what it is and focus on our strengths, talents, gifts and previous successes through adversity and take on the role as our very own personal coach. Then, like Novak, we give ourselves the opportunity to become 83.3 per cent more successful in overcoming the obstacles that we face at any given moment in our lives.

The power of self-dialogue as a metacognition tool cannot be underestimated and is well-supported in the research literature.[1] Naturally, there is a time and a place for these all-important conversations with ourselves. It is probably not the best idea to chat to yourself while shopping for groceries or grabbing a coffee!

DYNAMIC GOAL SETTING

Another metacognition strategy used by the world's best athletes is maintaining strong goal orientation. In professional sport, all great athletes are aligned to the same goal – to fulfil their own potential. Of course, the Olympics, World Cups, Grand Slams and endorsements fall into their set of aspirations, but self-improvement is always the primary drive.

The challenge with COVID-19, 4IR and the war in the Ukraine as a combined set is that they have the potential to strip all of us of our goals, dreams and aspirations. In such a climate of adversity, whether presenting as financial struggles, professional transitions, stormy relationships, family or health issues or any combination of stress, all goals seem to fade, only to be replaced with a central focus – survival!

Tony Robbins, an incredibly successful life and business strategist who has been at the top of his game for nearly four and a half decades, asserts that in order for us to experience joy and fulfilment, we need to feel that we are progressing in life. By this, I mean growing in a direction that is important to us (i.e. health and fitness, relationships, wealth, business, creative pursuits) each and every day, in a goal-orientated manner. Our happiness and purpose is dependent on this movement and Olympic champions never lose sight of this.

Yes, adversity does interfere with plans, schedules and preconstructed agendas, but it doesn't, nor should it, strip us of our desire for growth, aspirations and dreams. In these moments, we are called upon to strengthen our resolve and simply adjust, adapt, recalibrate, re-evaluate and repurpose our goals in real time.

MENTAL IMAGERY

The use of imagery is one of the most popular and well-accepted sport psychology strategies. It is used to improve performance, enhance coping mechanisms and to help recover from failures, disappointments and setbacks. Imagery is a mental process that can be practised and continually refined. At its core, it involves the creation and/or recreation of an experience.

Mental imagery allows us to step in and out of our past and futures on our terms. It also enables us to interpret the challenging events that we experience with more adaptability and greater agility, which supports planning and decision-making. For example, if you are experiencing health issues, visualising yourself recovered, fit and healthy will inspire you to make better choices pertaining to your healing. This could include improved food selection, increased (but measured) activity, nutritional supplements and better control within your immediate environment. Proper application of mental imagery replaces the fear of uncertainty with action and ultimately supports the realisation of the end goal.

Another good example is when preparing for a big presentation. Mentally rehearsing the delivery, picturing the audience, the lights, the atmosphere and the post-session questions will support a better delivery on the day. In many respects, you have already been there by creating a familiarity and, with that, a greater probability of success.

Our working memory[2] and future possibilities[3] are both supported and enhanced by the powerful mental exercise of imagery. Imagining a desired future not only supports us in the realisation of a dream, it also helps us better recall past experiences.

A 2020 meta-analysis of 55 high-quality studies, involving 1,438 athletes, showed that the practice of mental imagery not only enhances performance but also positively influences long-term results.[4] However, the German team of researchers also concluded that like most positive habits, the outcome is commensurate with the degree of effort put in.

Michael Phelps, the most successful and most decorated Olympians of all time, with a total 23 gold medals, began using mental imagery when he was a boy to calm his nerves and to help him focus. Mental imagery soon became one of his greatest weapons in and out of competition. According to Phelps: "When I would visualise, it would be what you want it to be, what you don't want it to be, what it could be. You are always ready for what comes your way."

At the Beijing Olympics in 2008, Phelps set himself a goal – to surpass Mark Spitz's record of winning seven gold medals in a single Olympic Games. Phelps was going to compete in eight events to break Spitz's long-standing record, held for 36 years, and would have to win a gold medal in every event and complete 17 races over nine days.

The feat would be nothing short of superhuman and, unlike Spitz who only swam 100- and 200-metre distances in two strokes (butterfly and freestyle), Phelps chose to compete across distances ranging from 100–400 metres and in all four strokes (breaststroke, backstroke, butterfly and freestyle).

Despite their admiration for Phelps, the swimming community believed his dream to be unattainable. Ian Thorpe, triple gold medallist at the games in Sydney in 2000, was vocal in expressing the impossibility, which further fuelled Michael's lofty ambitions.

Phelps' first event was the 400-metre medley in all four strokes. Not only did he win the gold in the event, he also set a new world record. In his next event, the 4 x 100-metre freestyle relay, he comfortably won his second gold and set yet another world record in the process. Then came the 200-metre freestyle and yet another gold, together with a new world record. Phelps seemed to be well on his way to rewriting the record books.

His next event was the one the swimming world and its fans had been waiting for. It was Michael's signature event – the 200-metre butterfly. The race began, Michael entered the water and his goggles came loose, quickly filling with water. By the time he crossed the 25-metre point he couldn't see a thing, he was swimming blind. For any other swimmer, their race would have been over. But not Michael Phelps.

He had prepared for the exact scenario through ongoing visualisation training throughout his career. In his mind, he had been there before and knew precisely what he needed to do. For the next 175 metres of the race, arguably the most physical and taxing portion of the event in the sport of swimming, Michael relied not on sight but rather on stroke count. Phelps was well aware of how many strokes he took in his first, second, third and fourth length in order to achieve his desired time. In one of the most spectacular outcomes in sporting history, Michael won the gold and broke the world record! The confidence that came from overcoming this seemingly insurmountable challenge saw Phelps go on to break another record and win gold in the 4 x 200-metre freestyle relay less than 30 minutes later.

Six gold and six world records later, Michael faced the second great challenge of the games – Milorad Čavić, the 100-metre butterfly specialist. Michael started the race poorly, coming in seventh at the 50-metre turn. However, he was somehow able to come back over the next 50 metres to win the race by the smallest margin in swimming history – 0.01 seconds. He had matched Mark Spitz's record and silenced the critics.

In the final race, the 4 x 100-metre medley, Michael and his Team USA teammates Brendan Hansen, Aaron Peirsol and Jason Lezak smashed the world record, giving Phelps his eighth gold medal and seventh Olympic record, something that is unlikely to ever be achieved again in the world of sport.

Another iconic athlete, Michael Jordan, was a big proponent of visualisation and used it throughout his sensational career. According to Jordan: "I trained my mind vigorously to visualise an image of the basketball going through the hoop. Eventually it became a seamless difference between my imagination and reality."

The list of top performers who draw on this powerful metacognition skill is endless.

There is no doubt that mental imagery, when deliberate, practised regularly and used strategically, can inspire us to push through all the setbacks, limitations and barriers that clutter our lives. Moreover, imagery will support self-confidence and even help place us in a success-orientated mindset.

Most of us do already use mental imagery when encountering adversity but, instead of using it to create a vision or story of the future we want, we tend to create an array of negative scenarios. Catastrophising is all too common in a world fraught with hypervigilance. When business is slow, we have visions of not being able to pay the bills. When we experience conflict in the home, visions of months of couples therapy or even a potential divorce can dominate. And of course the most common scenario during the COVID-19 pandemic – the sore throat or tight chest. Any degree of irritability or compromise in those areas immediately drew images of COVID-19, isolation and a team of specialists around us in full protective gear.

The lesson here is simple – when we experience challenges, change, uncertainty, hardships and setbacks, we would be well-served to draw on the skills and habits used by Olympic champions and elite athletes. One of these psychological strategies requires that we make a conscious decision to see the future we want and not the one we fear. It is important to remind ourselves that mental imagery is a skill. It may start off as being difficult and challenging, but the more we practise, the more often we repeat it, the better we will become.

■

CONTROL YOUR STRESS RESPONSES

Adversity, regardless of intensity, frequency or duration will evoke the stress axis. Olympic champions, like all of us, constantly experience overwhelming stress to the extent that it affects every aspect of their wellbeing. What separates them from everyone else is that they are able to control the stress axis (and associated biological responses) exceptionally well. Within the context of resilience and the realisation of one's fullest potential, this skill is all-important.

The destructive force of chronic stress is known to all of us, but what is less well understood is that there are many barriers to proper stress regulation that affect many of us. As mentioned in Part 1, this includes a childhood history of physical or emotional abuse, trauma, neglect, uncertainty or living in a state of constant fear.

These experiences can manifest in disproportional stress responses (specifically in the case of physical abuse and trauma), heightened stress reactivity (when growing up in a state of constant threat) or an inability to regulate stress responses (driven principally by neglect and emotional abuse). Sadly, many people are subjected to a combination of these adversities throughout the course of their childhood. At the same time, inherited genetic polymorphisms, specifically relating to FKBP5 (which is associated with the inability to properly shut down the stress response), CRHR1 (which is linked to an increased severity of our physiological response to stress) and many of the serotonin-related genes can further amplify stress reactions and/or result in a complete failure to regulate stress responses following a stressful experience.

One of the most profound metacognition skills seen in Olympians is the ability to quickly identify at what point their stress axis and cortisol have become chronically elevated or alternatively raised to the extent that it is overwhelming their intrinsic coping mechanisms. More importantly, once recognised (either through tracking devises that measure sleep, heart rate variability [HRV] and resting heart or subjective experience), they are consciously able to shut down the stress axis and create biological stability before it negatively impacts their health (mental and physical), adaptability and performance.

Michael Phelps, Cristiano Ronaldo and Novak Djokovic all cite stress-reduction techniques as contributing to their incredible career success and longevity.

Regulation and control over the stress axis can be achieved through many different pathways, including social buffering, drawing strongly on social support and connection, meditation or selecting behaviours that target the release of oxytocin (for example, taking vitamin C, magnesium L-threonate and quercetin, aerobic exercise, music therapy), which is known to directly inhibit the stress response.

However, when it comes to stress axis mastery – the ability to turn stress off at will – all paths will ultimately converge on some form of controlled breathing, whether it is practised as a standalone or as part of meditation, yoga or even aquatic routine.

Breathing, together with heart rate and other vital functions, is governed by a small region of the brain known as the brainstem. Despite making up only 2.6 per cent of the brain's total weight, the brainstem not only governs some of the most essential life-sustaining functions, it is also the point of origin for many influential nerves, including the master regulator of stress, cardiorespiratory, hormonal and immune behaviours[5] – the vagus nerve.

The brainstem does more than simply determine the rate of inspiration and expiration; it also influences the type of breath we need to take.

Regular breaths, sighs, yawns, sniffs, coughs, laughs and cries all have their own unique signature and influence on our wellbeing. The rate and type of breath we take is constantly matched to our immediate environment, physiological state, psychological experiences and perceptions.

In order to determine what kind of breath we need to take, the brainstem gathers information from its resident chemoreceptors (super specialised sensors) to ascertain the current levels of oxygen (O_2), carbon dioxide (CO_2) and pH (a quantitative measure of acidity) within the surrounding fluid. It also receives information from remote sensors located within the heart and carotid artery in front of the neck, together with hyper-sensitive pressure receptors located within the lungs. It is an astounding feat of information processing and reactive measures.

One of the most important subconscious life-sustaining reflexes driven by the brainstem is the physiological sigh. A sigh is an involuntary deep breath that starts out normally, but before you exhale, you take a second even larger breath and then pause briefly before breathing out.

> The sigh involves two staggered inhales, followed by a long exhale.

In other words, you double inhale, pause and exhale. A sigh increases breathing volume by anything from 200 per cent to 500 per cent and occurs without any conscious thought every 5 minutes or so.[6]

Scientists have determined that the primary purpose of sighing is to re-inflate the half a billion tiny, delicate, balloon-like sacs in the lungs called alveoli. The alveoli are where O_2 enters and CO_2 leaves the bloodstream. What tends to happen during the normal breathing process is that the tiny air sacs spontaneously collapse over a period of minutes, causing increased lung resistance, decreased lung compliance (elasticity) and a potential build-up of carbon dioxide.

At this point, you might be wondering how this deep dive into physiology is relevant to resilience, performance, stress and managing a state of over-arousal. The answer lies with CO_2.

Research shows that an excessive build-up of CO_2 will trigger stress responses and cause elevated cortisol levels.[7] This can be a consequence of several emotional, physical and environmental factors, which include worry, anxiety, underlying medical conditions (especially pertaining to the respiratory system), an infection (viral or bacterial), smoking or air pollution. The effect is so pronounced that a single inhalation of air that consists of 35 per cent CO_2 is a medical assessment that is gaining popularity as a vulnerability and predictability measure for current and future stress-related disorders. Research shows that individuals with an underlying panic disorder who experience social phobias, general anxiety disorder or who are prone to PTSD will display greater reactivity to the test.[8]

This scientific principle is something that I have lived with and experienced on many occasions. Several years ago I sustained a knee injury due to some rather over-zealous training and took up swimming during the long and painstaking recovery period. Not a particularly good swimmer at the time (in fact I was nothing short of terrible), I decided to enlist the services of a professional swimming coach to help me with my overall technique. One of the many challenges I had in the early learning stages, related to my breathing, specifically related to poor efficiency, which limited my swimming endurance.

Included in the coach's training and development process were drills referred to as "hypoxic exercises". While this form of swimming training does involve some breath-holding (25–50 metres under water or whatever one's tolerance allowed), the focus is more orientated to reduced breathing frequency while swimming. As an example, for one length I would perform ten freestyle strokes to a single breath, the next length would be eight, then six until one reaches a ratio of two to one.

There are no words to describe the degree of panic and anxiety I used to experience during these sets – they were horrible and it had nothing to do with the physical exertion and everything to do with the build up of CO_2. To my surprise at the time, not every member of the swimming group experienced the same degree of stress in response to these drills.

Clearly I fell into a more vulnerable group, being predisposed to anxiety in its many forms and expressions. Many competitive swimmers are all too familiar with dramatically elevated levels of CO_2 and the resulting psychological effect.

With this understanding of the role of CO_2 in stress axis activation or amplification, we can appreciate the importance and relevance of the physiological sigh. Incredibly, by consciously sighing we have the power to deliberately reduce CO_2 levels and instantaneously reduce stress.

This simple technique can help maintain optimal levels of arousal and emotional stability under acute challenging conditions. Whether you are in a heated meeting, delivering a presentation to an overly critical audience, playing in a tight match or perhaps the toughest challenge of them all – when your three-year-old has a meltdown when you suggest he takes off his superhero suit he has been wearing for the last seven days. This simple breath sequence can help with all-important momentary composure.

Several studies done on anxious individuals show some astonishing findings on this ancient reflex of sighing, including improved balance within the nervous system, a dramatic reduction in muscle tension and a prevailing sense of relief.[9]

While a sigh offers a practical short-term solution of about 5 minutes to the immediate challenges that confront us, the bigger picture within the context of stress axis regulation and resilience is unquestionably slow breathing techniques. Slow breathing techniques involve less than 10 breaths a minute, which is considerably less than normal breathing at rest (12–18 breaths per minute) and most certainly during activity (40–60 breaths per minute).

Stefanos Tsitsipas is one of the most exciting tennis players in recent years, with one of the best forehands in the history of the sport. By the age of 23, he was already ranked 3 in the world, pushing aside the likes of Nadal, Djokovic and Federer. While his forehand is an obvious weapon, by his admission, his secret weapon (and now no longer a secret) is better breathing!

Following a big title win, Tsitsipas talked about breathing and its impact on his growing success. "I find breathing very important. Breathing is something I've been working on for the last couple of months with my psychologist. Especially when I'm performing or playing, breathing helps me control myself and have full control of what I'm doing out there. When you breathe well, I feel like your game is capable of reaching the top."[10]

In order to derive the maximum physical and emotional benefit from slow breathing techniques, we need to reduce our frequency of breaths to 5–6 breaths per minute (10–12 seconds per breath). This slow rate of respiration is associated with a significant activation and strengthening of the vagus nerve.

A 2018 meta-analysis with a title that reads more like a statement, "How Breath-Control Can Change Your Life: A Systematic Review on Psycho-Physiological Correlates of Slow Breathing", showed that taking 5–6 breaths a minute for a sustained period (i.e. several minutes) is associated with reduced anxiety, fear and anger as well as improved relaxation and a more positive mindset.[11] This emotional influence is a result of several factors, including a distinct alteration in brain wave patterns favouring an alpha state, which is associated with calmness and restful alertness. Another contributing factor in emotional regulation is the increased activation of the default mode network (DMN), which strongly supports better imagination, creativity and cognition. Finally, the review also showed that slow breathing techniques induce a greater supply of oxygenated blood to the brain's resilience epicentres, including the prefrontal cortex.

The physical effects are equally impressive and cannot be disentangled from the positive emotional and psychological shifts. By stimulating the vagus nerve and improving the strength of its influence over the parasympathetic nervous system (the network of nerves that relaxes our body), we are able to better support physical recovery and regeneration, relaxation, optimal immune and hormonal behaviours and overall biological balance.

The primary measure of vagus nerve integrity is HRV. HRV has a profound influence on resilience and adaptability and is the physiological phenomenon of the variation in the time interval between consecutive heartbeats measured in milliseconds. Although it may seem counter-intuitive, a healthy, non-stressed heart does not beat like a metronome. Instead, when observing the timing between heartbeats, there is constant variation. This variation indicates that our nervous system is able to optimally adjust and adapt to changes within our biological state.

Imagine you are sitting in a comfortable chair at home reading a book. While immersed in the experience, your heart is beating at 60 beats per minute. At 60 beats per minute, your heart is contracting at a rate of one beat per second. However, only under stressful conditions, general fatigue or in a compromised state of health would your heart behave in this predicable fashion. In fact, what is actually taking place while you are sitting and reading is shorter and longer periods between heartbeats based on exquisite internal feedback, your immediate psychological state, the environmental conditions and, of course, the integrity and strength of the vagus nerve. This entire process can be seen as an ultra-sensitive biological calibrator. The better you can adjust physiologically speaking, the higher your HRV is likely to be, and the better you will adapt in times of adversity.

HRV is recognised as a primary indicator for individual physical conditioning, general health and reactivity to and recovery from stress. Moreover, higher HRV is associated with exceptional stress regulation, robust health, improved cognition and a lower overall risk of disease.[12] In addition to its psychological and physical health benefits, what makes HRV so valuable from a resilience standpoint is that it is easily measured with health and fitness trackers, such as rings, wrist or chest straps.

The table on p.187 offers simple and practical tools to support better control and regulation of stress responses. Bear in mind that any one or

Stress management tools and techniques

Activity	How it works to reduce stress/arousal	Method/s	Suggested application	Number of repetitions/ or duration	Best practice and environment
The physi-ological sigh	Rapid reduction in carbon dioxide levels	Double inhale, pause, exhale (second inhale is greater than first)	During periods of acute over-arousal/ stress	2–3	In the situation itself (i.e. at your desk, on the court, before giving a presentation, etc.)
Slow, controlled breathing	Activation and strengthening of the vagus nerve, increased activity in the brain's executive regions, alpha brain waves state, increased activation of DMN	Inhale: 4 secs Exhale: 6 secs Inhale: 5.5 secs Exhale: 5.5 secs Inhale: 6 secs Exhale: 6 secs	Daily practice, especially during periods that are more stressful and/ or when feeling dysregulated	2–15 mins	Find a quiet place where you won't be interrupted. You can either sit upright or lie down. Slow your breathing rate down to the desired rate. Be sure to inhale through your nose and exhale through your mouth. The deep inhalation should cause the ribs to expand and the abdomen to rise.
Meditation	Activation and strengthening of the vagus nerve, increased recruit-ment and activity in the brain's execu-tive regions, reduced activity in the brain's stress and fear processing areas	Focused-based Open-monitoring Mindfulness-based stress reduction Loving kindness	Daily practice, especially during periods that are more stressful and/ or when feeling dysregulated	12–60 mins	Find a quiet space where you can sit or lie down. If you lack meditation experience or training, it may be advantageous to find a practitioner or download one of the many apps that are available.
Mind/body exercises	Activation and strengthening of the vagus nerve	Yoga Tai chi Qigong	Several times a week or as time or budget allows	10–60 mins	Proper technique and an emphasis on breath is important, as is proper instruction
Swimming or aquatic activities	Vagus nerve activation mediated by the dive reflex	All strokes that favour short-term head submergence	It is particularly effective on days when feeling overwhelmed	15–45 mins	Unless you have previous training or experience, consider instruction/coaching to assist with breathing (and stroke) technique

combination of these activities will promote improved cardiovascular health, reduce inflammation, enhance physical and mental health and increase cognitive performance and creativity.[13] I suggest interchanging these modalities based on your current state of health, time availability, access to service providers and/or equipment.

In itself, the combination of cognitive reappraisal (seeing stresses as providing opportunities for growth, development and mastery) and metacognition (the use of goal setting, imagery, self-talk and stress-response regulation) offers an incredible framework for resilience, but there is more to the story.

The landmark study done by Fletcher and Sarkar on the group of Olympic champions also uncovered that these athletes possess the ability to utilise and augment a constellation of additional psychological characteristics and factors to withstand adversity and challenge. The primary traits were positive personality, motivation, confidence, focus and drawing on social support. Exploring these psychological features and how we can effectively apply them to our own lives and challenges is covered in the upcoming section.

■

SECTION SUMMARY

- Metacognition is an exceptionally powerful resilience trait. Metacognition is the ability to understand and control one's own thoughts and is dependent on self-awareness and self-mastery.
- This resilience skill encompasses positive self-dialogue, goal setting, the use of mental imagery and the conscious and deliberate manipulation of levels of arousal.
- A strong commitment to goal setting, pursuit and realisation supports resilience.

- Mental imagery is a popular and well-accepted sport psychology strategy that is used to improve performance, enhance coping mechanisms and recover from failures, disappointments and setbacks.
- By controlling our stress responses, we are able to gain better control over our emotional state and overall mental health.
- Like Olympic champions, we need to be better able to rapidly recognise a state of over-arousal and/or stress axis dysfunction and then consciously regulate ourselves. With this self-awareness, we are able to rapidly mitigate any negative impacts of chronic stress and strain.
- Controlled breathing is one of the most effective ways of managing stress and feelings of being overwhelmed.
- The physiological sigh is one of the most important life-sustaining reflexes. The primary purpose of the sigh is to maintain lung function and integrity as well as rid the body of excess carbon dioxide (a known stress trigger).
- Not only does a sigh remove excess carbon dioxide from our body, but it also improves balance within our nervous system, reduces muscle tension and promotes emotional discharge.
- Slow controlled breathing techniques (under 10 breaths a minute) are a strong stimulus for the vagus nerve.
- Performing 5–6 breaths per minute for a sustained period is associated with reduced anxiety, fear and anger as well as improved relaxation and a more positive mindset.
- The combination of cognitive reappraisal and metacognition (i.e. self-dialogue, mental imagery, stress regulation and goal setting) offers an exceptional framework for resilience promotion and development.

POSITIVE PERSONALITY

When people see your personality come out, they feel so good,
like they actually know who you are.

USAIN BOLT

Much like those individuals who are inherently resilient in the face of adversity, Olympic champions exhibit a wide range of positive personality traits, including extroversion, openness to new experiences, conscientiousness, optimism, adaptive perfectionism and proactivity. Not all champions possess all of these traits and, as with many human characteristics, there will always be individual strengths and vulnerabilities. If we wish to successfully apply the learnings that follow to our own lives, the best place to start is by building on the traits we are most comfortable with and that come easily to us. We then slowly and systematically open ourselves up to exploring and developing those traits that we have historically shied away from.

Don't be afraid to break out of your shell.

SPORT'S GREATEST SHOWMAN

No athlete knows just how to "wow" the crowd like the larger-than-life sprint legend Usain Bolt. His superhuman achievements parallel his effervescent personality. Bolt is known for his enthusiasm in taking photos with fans, dancing or singing during TV appearances and interviews, fist-pumping officials or performing a humorous antic that has the stadium and viewers laughing and applauding.

On the business end, Bolt holds the world record in the 100 metres (9.58 seconds), 200 metres (19.19 seconds) and the 4 x 100-metre relay (37.10 seconds). He also achieved the impossible by winning the gold medal in the 100 and 200 metres in three consecutive Olympics (Beijing 2008, London 2012 and Rio 2016). Bolt's sprint performances are so ahead of our time that when Ethan Segal, a theoretical astrophysicist at Lewis & Clark College, charted a graph looking at the incremental progression of the 100-metre world record over the past 100 years, he discovered that in terms of speed over 100 and 200 metres, Bolt is performing at a level approximately 30 years beyond that of the expected capabilities of modern man. Mathematically, Bolt belongs at the 2040 Olympics or beyond.

Bolt's extroverted persona could fool us into believing that his journey to stardom was effortless and merely a product of gifted genetics and perfect upbringing. But this is not the case. The reality is that Usain Bolt suffers from severe scoliosis. Scoliosis is a sideways curvature of the spine and is associated with excruciating back pain, spasms, inflammation, reduced range of motion and pelvic issues that are negatively associated with walking and running.

Bolt's scoliosis is so severe (more than a 40-degree curvature) that his right leg is a full 11 millimetres shorter than his left. As a consequence, Bolt's sprint technique is hugely asymmetrical, creating significantly higher loads on his right side. Whether or not this gives Bolt some sort of advantage in speed and performance is unclear (and highly unlikely), but what is certain is that this disparity is associated with an extremely high prevalence of injuries, especially in the lower extremities (hamstrings and calves) and back. Not surprisingly, Bolt's career has been dominated by reoccurring injuries, placing constant pressure on his endorsements, earning potential and career longevity. This was immediately apparent from 2004, the year he turned professional. During his first Olympics, Bolt was eliminated in his first round due to a hamstring injury. It was a disappointing and frustrating start as a professional athlete. Even during the final race of Bolt's career at the 2017 World Championships in London, Bolt collapsed on the track, clutching his hamstring in the 4 x 100-metre relay event. Yet, despite the setbacks, the many disappointments, missed opportunities and repeated failures – when it mattered, when the stakes were at the highest possible level and the pressure was at full throttle – he was able to unleash superhuman performances.

Bolt is the quintessential extrovert and in many respects this is his resilience superpower. He is fuelled by performing in front of large expectant crowds, bright lights, cameras, frenzied media and, of course, fierce and combative opponents. While many would break under the pressure, to him the pressure and tension is pure oxygen – his life force. His competitive advantage at the Olympics is the occasion itself.

Usain Bolt's story highlights the immense value of extroversion, optimism and positivity in overcoming life's many hurdles. Yet, for many, myself included, extroversion is neither a natural disposition nor a comfortable experience.

Over the years, scientists have proposed several theories as to why some people are more extroverted than others. What some research shows is that more *introverted* personalities may have raised levels of arousal in the brain's executive regions, making any additional stimulus (of all types) feel overwhelming and unsettling.[1] In a sense, introverted personalities may shy away from crowds and bustling activities to prevent the experience of over-arousal.

Another well-supported model shows that *extroverted* personalities have heightened sensitivity and reactivity to dopamine which may drive them to behaviours or activities that increase this powerful neurotransmitter.[2]

Finally, it has also been suggested that there may even be differences in neurochemical affinity among individuals where extroverts are driven by increased dopamine activity, whereas introverts will favour acetylcholine, which, like dopamine, also supports memory, attention and cognition but has additional balancing effects within the brain.[3]

Although there is still much to learn about extroversion, what we need to realise is that while genetics do account for 40–60 per cent of our more prominent personality traits, the environment we grow up in, and then later create for ourselves, is equally as impactful and in some instances even more so.[4] In other words, we have the power to choose who and what we want to be, including being more outgoing and expressive. It may take an accompaniment of soothing techniques (breathing and meditation) and brief time-outs throughout the course of the day, but we can all shatter our self-imposed shells should we want to, or need to, because life demands this of us.

Throughout my childhood and young adulthood, I was petrified of speaking in front of people. This fear was so great that I would consider a group to be two or more individuals. When speaking to an audience, I would become shaky, largely incoherent and completely overwhelmed. As time passed and I moved into different roles in my professional career, speaking to audiences became a central feature and expectation of my work. For the first few years (or even decades), I was still overwhelmed by the experience and would not sleep the night before an event. Fortunately, I always loved the content of my presentations and once I had overcome those initial nerves (which could take 30 minutes or longer) I would settle down. Fast-forward to today and public speaking has become my primary job. I love it, I thrive under the pressure, I enjoy large audiences, the lights, the noise, the attention and the energy. I do still need a few periods in my day to destress and, when the opportunity arises, I take a 10–15-minute nap, but my professional environment has transformed me into – dare I say – an extrovert.

We need to always be mindful that enhancing any personality characteristic, including extroversion, takes work, effort and time. To make the resilience journey easier, it is advantageous to leverage off those positive personality traits (i.e. extroversion, an openness to new experiences, conscientiousness, optimism, adaptive perfectionism and proactivity) that come more naturally.

When it comes to personal growth and development, addressing our inherent weaknesses and limitations is important, but it is equally important to further develop and amplify our existing strengths.

OPENNESS TO NEW EXPERIENCES

The COVID-19 pandemic evoked varied experiences and responses for people. For most, it was a waiting period for when things were expected to return to "normal". Millions around the world resisted the change and clung on to pre-existing views of life pertaining to relationships, business, hobbies and politics. For many people, it was a frustrating and painful time, as it has translated into a long holding pattern of stagnation and waiting. Not moving forward, growing and evolving is associated with reduced joy, happiness, fulfilment and purpose in life.

By contrast, there were other people who accepted change as a reality, the past as a bygone era and the future as offering new possibilities – despite the short-term burdens, restrictions and challenges. They used the time to upskill, learn, develop their creative side, get fit, savour the additional time with their family and prepare themselves for an unknown future. Despite the fears and uncertainty, they had hope. It is this openness to new realities and possibilities that drives resilience and reduces vulnerability to adversity.

As a human trait, openness is complex and has many layers and should not be confused with being easy-going and accommodating. Rather, openness brings imagination, feelings, ideas, values and aesthetics, together with intelligence, resourcefulness, competence, introspection and reflection.[5] At the same time, it demands intellectual curiosity, interests, emotional richness and unconventionality.

Studies have identified openness as a strong driver of all scales of creativity (the ability to think in a less linear and more elastic fashion) and it is even recognised as a measure of creative potential.[6] In fact, of the positive personality traits (i.e. extroversion, openness, conscientiousness, optimism, adaptive perfectionism and proactivity), openness is the only one to show direct associations with creativity. A 2016 study found that openness is not only associated with but also highly predictive of creative achievements.[7] The association between openness and creativity (especially divergent thinking) and resilience is so strong that researchers suggest it may even be a predictive measure. In other words, if you are creative and open, you are resilient.

> Being open requires that you are curious, imaginative, competent, resourceful, reflective and have the courage to be a little unconventional.

This does makes sense as openness and creativity offer us something quite unique in adversity. Not only does creativity help us to generate and act on positive solutions in the face of stress, challenges and uncertainty, it also allows us to be optimistic and reality bound, logical and naïve and introverted or extroverted, based on the situation we find ourselves in.

The quick self-assessment on p.195 will give you a basic idea as to your current level of openness.

Scoring
Very open to new experiences: 16–24 points
In the middle of the openness spectrum: 8–16 points
Low on the openness front (for now):   0–8 points

No matter where you scored on this assessment, openness and creativity is something that can be developed. Research shows that the genetic contribution to the experience of openness is a mere 21 per cent.

Openness self-assessment

Openness avenues	Yes, definitely (3 points)	Sometimes (2 points)	Seldom (1 point)
I can see possibilities that aren't always obvious to others in a given situation			
I try to understand the deeper meanings and/or concepts behind events			
Understanding the mechanism as to how things work is important to me			
I need some sort of creative outlet in my life			
My imagination can be very active at times			
I enjoy exploring new places, cultures and environments			
I place a high value on aesthetics and artistry			
I prefer to discuss complex theories and deep concepts as opposed to engaging in small talk			

PROMOTING OPENNESS AND CREATIVITY

Contrary to the popular view that creativity doesn't require conscious effort and occurs somewhat spontaneously, a study done in 2008 by Dutch researchers from the University of Amsterdam proposed that creativity and openness are under the direct influence of two very distinctive and elective psychological processes.[8]

- Cognitive flexibility (the level of ease with which we can switch to a different approach or consider a different perspective)

■ Cognitive persistence (the degree of sustained and focused effort that can be applied to a challenge or given situation).

This understanding implies that for us to be more creative and open to new realities, we need to be flexible enough to switch between interests, approaches, notions, concepts and experiences. At the same time, we need to be prepared to work on creative solutions in a way that is system-, process- and effort-driven.

Both cognitive flexibility and persistence are directly affected by our perceptions of stress and our current emotional state. The Dutch researchers published a meta-analysis examining 25 years of research in the area of creativity. What the study showed was that the more activating positive mood states, such as excitement, joy and happiness, significantly enhance creativity and promote the experience of openness.[9] At the same time, the review identified that chronic stress, depression, anxiety, worry, irritability and sadness have an adverse effect on creativity. This challenges the common perceptions that originality, cognitive flexibility and thought fluency are acquired when we struggle within, i.e. the struggling artist analogy.

An important topic within the framework of creativity is the relationship between anxiety (generalised, social phobias, obsessive-compulsive disorder, panic disorder or post-traumatic stress disorder) and openness. What makes this relationship so relevant is that anxiety ranks as one of the leading disease burdens globally.[10] Moreover, since the outbreak of COVID-19, there has been a 25.6 per cent spike in anxiety-based disorders globally.[11]

In an analysis of 59 studies within the review, it was shown that anxiety is significantly and negatively associated with creative performance.[12] In other words, if you are experiencing anxiety in any way, shape or form, it becomes extremely difficult to solve problems and find creative solutions.

This begs the question – how does someone become more "open" in a world besieged by chronic stress and uncertainty? It appears somewhat conflicting that in order to successfully cope with adversity and change, we require openness and creativity, yet, under conditions of chronic stress, worry and anxiety, this key resilience trait is impaired.

In 2013 a team of researchers from Singapore Management University published a study that was able to shed light on this apparent paradox.[13] What the study identified and presented so eloquently was that there is a dance – a dynamic interplay of sorts – between negative and positive emotional states that best support openness and creative processes. This model shows that creativity is significantly increased when we first experience stress, adversity, a setback or a failure. Then, following the challenging event, we are plunged into a positive environment where we can transform fear into enthusiasm, excitement, happiness and joy.

The advantage of the initial challenge is that it is able to achieve a narrowing of attentional focus, drawing awareness to existing problems and signalling to us that effort is required. At the same time, a stressful event can serve as an incubator for new ideas that will emerge later on when we are placed in a supportive and uplifting environment. The simple message here is that adversity can be an incredible catalyst for innovation

Optimising creativity and innovation

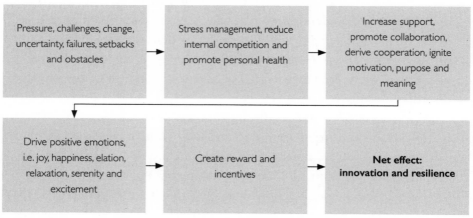

and creativity, but only if you are able to rapidly and successfully create an environment of positivity and reduced stress in real time.

Although these aspects are beyond the scope of this book, it is important to mention that other important creativity drivers include cooperation (as opposed to competition)[14] and reward and, as such, can and should be used to bring both our own as well as others' potential to life.

THE NEUROBIOLOGICAL DRIVERS OF CREATIVITY

Like many resilience traits, openness is driven largely by the executive regions of the brain (specifically the prefrontal cortex),[15] the default mode network (DMN) as well as several neurochemicals, namely dopamine, norephedrine and serotonin.[16] Although openness has several neurochemical influences, dopamine appears to be the biggest driver in this regard. Neuroscientists have identified two clear pathways through which dopamine promotes openness, creativity and innovative potential.

The first pathway is known as the mesocortical pathway and it supports and promotes dopamine activity within the brain's executive regions. This enhances working memory, conscious shifting of thoughts and filtering of perceivably irrelevant influences. The second is known as the nigrostriatal pathway and supports and increases dopamine activity in a region of the brain known as the striatum. Striatal dopamine augments creative drives, mood, emotion and motivation. This duality of dopamine broadcasting supports flexibility and persistence in our creative pursuits. Without at least moderate levels of dopamine, creativity and openness simply can't exist.[17]

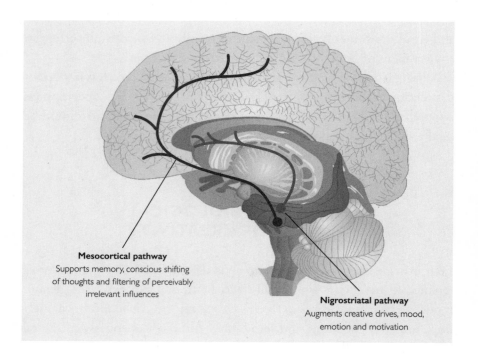

Mesocortical pathway
Supports memory, conscious shifting
of thoughts and filtering of perceivably
irrelevant influences

Nigrostriatal pathway
Augments creative drives, mood,
emotion and motivation

Dopamine – is it nature or nurture?

Genetics have a profound influence on resilience. However, when it comes to the dopaminergic system, while genetics do influence dopamine synthesis, transport and recollection (especially the DAT gene), uptake and signalling within nerve cells (most notably the DRD4 and DRD2 genes) or overall metabolism and breakdown (COMT) and may predispose individuals to vulnerability, it should be noted that if inherited variants exist they can be minimised, nullified or positively transformed by the environment we choose to create for ourselves.

The dopamine system can be further divided into baseline levels (tonic) that continuously circulate and peak (phasic) during very specific activities (for example, scanning social media). For us to promote resilience, our goal should be to influence baseline levels and not pursue the peaks through pharmaceutical agents (unless medically indicated) or other behaviours (i.e. social media, internet addiction, gambling, etc.).

The table on these pages highlights some of the more effective and healthy ways to raise baseline dopamine levels, improve transport and reuptake, augment signalling and support dopamine metabolism. Because dopamine underpins most resilience behaviours, these methods can offer tremendous support in times of adversity.

Dopamine toolkit

Activity	Effect	Application	Special considerations
Cold immersion (cold baths, cold showers, ice soaks, going outside on a very cold day, cryotherapy chamber)	Can achieve a 250% increase in dopamine, which is sustained for prolonged periods of time (over three hours)	Water-based immersion **Total weekly exposure:** 11 mins or slightly more per week **Temperature ranges:** 8–15 °C (experienced individuals can reduce this slightly if desired) **Time range:** 3–20 mins **Suggested:** Ice baths for 3 mins × 3 sets (with 2–3 min break) or 9 mins continuous (8–12 °C)	NB: Consult with your doctor before trying any cold-immersion protocol, as it affects blood pressure, heart rate and circulation. Moreover, it can cause significant heart stress.
Aerobic exercise	Raises dopamine by up to 200%, largely through the increased expression of an enzyme (tyrosine hydroxylase), which helps convert tyrosine (a protein) into dopamine. Exercise also improves dopamine signalling (through receptor binding), meaning that dopamine's effects are more magnified. Finally, exercise supports and protects the dopamine-producing cells.	**Minimum duration:** 7–20 mins **Maximum duration:** Based on fitness and aspirations **Intensity:** Higher intensities (including HIIT) would theoretically evoke greater responses, due to BDNF being a dopamine protagonist	Higher levels of aerobic fitness are correlated to elevated baseline dopamine and greater cognition and resilience.

Activity	Effect	Application	Special considerations
Music	Enjoyable music can increase dopamine by 9% or more, especially if it produces chills. Also, pleasurable music is associated with increased blood flow and increased activation in the striatum, a region that drives creativity from a place of emotion, mood and motivation.	During periods when you require creative thinking, persistence and motivation, put on some of your favourite music.	Try not to stack too many dopamine-elevating activities on top of one another (i.e. music while having an ice bath), as it can result in diminishment of overall effects and a possible dopamine dip.
Sunlight exposure	Promotes increased dopamine signalling (greater D2 and D3 receptor concentration) in the region of the brain associated with creative drives.	**Minimum exposure:** 2–10 mins a day **Ideal exposure:** 10–30 mins **Optimal time:** First thing in the morning	Caution: It's generally recommended to limit sun exposure during peak hours when ultraviolet radiation is the strongest, typically between 9am and 3pm, and to apply sunscreen when the UV index is above 3.
Meditation	Meditation can be associated with a 65% increase in dopamine. However, for baseline levels to increase, meditation needs to be practised fairly regularly.	**Minimum duration:** 12–13 mins **Type:** Based on preference and method of instruction **Frequency:** Daily or every second day	A major benefit of meditation is that it is associated with greater activity in the regions of the brain that are associated with openness and creativity.
Massage, osteopathy and physical therapies	Physical therapies are associated with a 21–42% increase in dopamine.	**Duration:** 15–30 mins **Frequency:** Two or more times per week	Another benefit of physical therapies is that they are able to reduce cortisol, with research reporting a 23–45% reduction in adults.

CONSCIENTIOUSNESS – A REMARKABLE SKILLSET

Conscientiousness is a significant resilience factor and happens to be one of the most impactful of all the positive personality influences. Over and above the influence on resilience, conscientiousness is a strong negative predictor of disease risk throughout your lifespan. In other words, the more conscientious you are, the lower your risk of disease and premature mortality from all causes.[18]

This is not surprising when we consider the spectrum of habits and behaviours that make up conscientiousness, including being organised, planning ahead, effective goal setting and measured behaviours. At the same time, it also encompasses a commitment to hard work, personal growth and achievement, which is augmented by self-discipline and self-control. Moreover, conscientiousness is associated with a greater degree of personal responsibility, accountability, reliability and high values.

Conscientious behaviour is not without its challenges. Taken to the extreme, it can spark rigidity, inflexibility, perfectionism and overachiever-type behaviours, which may actually detract from resilience and increase vulnerability to adversity. As with so many habits, achieving a state of balance should always be the end goal. The checklist opposite might assist you to incorporate these components into your life. I have completed Monday's tasks as an example.

Over a period of more than two decades of living and working in professional sport, I have learnt a great deal from professional athletes and their teams – conscientiousness being one of the more prominent and ongoing lessons. Upon reflection, the greatest teachings in this area have centred around emotional regulation (something I am still trying to master), self-discipline and self-control.

The following chart offers the opportunity for deep self-reflection and a way of identifying areas of strength together with areas of opportunity from a conscientiousness standpoint. The self-rating scale ranges from 1 (poor) to 5 (exceptional). Where you have scores of 3 or below see these traits as levers that can be pulled to dramatically enhance your resilience potential. As with the quick assessment of page 37, perform the test with a close friend, family member or partner. Circle the number that best describes where you feel your level is and following this ask your partner to rate you objectively. Clarity always exists in the middle of the two ratings.

A conscientiousness snapshot

	1	2	3	4	5
I try to plan ahead where I can					
I am very detail orientated					
On the most part my life is structured					
I commit a certain portion of my day/week to self-improvement and personal growth					
I tend not to procrastinate or waste time					
I have a very strong value set which I seldom (if ever) compromise					

The following list of conscientiousness hacks is based on my experience with sports stars and their teams. In your personal resilience journey, developing one or more of the following traits can be immeasurably supportive:

- Be more prepared and plan ahead
- Place a stronger emphasis on the finer details, together with the broader strokes
- Create and promote more structure in your life
- Commit to self-improvement and continued growth
- Try to avoid procrastinating and/or time wastage
- Try to do what is right and not what is popular.

STRIVE TO BE MORE PROACTIVE

Olympic champions are not passive recipients of environmental constraints on their behaviours or actions. They constantly work and strive to intentionally transform their current performances and environment by proactively exploring better commercial opportunities, more innovative tools and products, advanced training methods as well as engaging with highly skilled practitioners around the world.

Olympic champions have complete confidence in their ability to transcend the restraints of situational forces and initiate positive changes regardless of their given environment and challenges. In other words, they strongly believe that they are not limited or constrained by their circumstances and, through their deliberate actions, they have the power to shape their world.

Proactivity is a force to be reckoned with. Having your sights on the future and being action-orientated is associated with tremendous success in life (and sport), regardless of challenges and adversity. A 2018 study focusing on creative behaviour, commitment and work performance found that when compared to passive individuals, proactive personalities are significantly more creative and show higher levels of overall performance in the workplace.[19]

In order to be proactive, you are required to be anticipatory (loads of experience certainly helps in this regard) as well as change- and action-orientated. One of the biggest realisations that stemmed from the COVID-19 pandemic was the devastating impact that dramatic and rapid change, together with ongoing uncertainty, can have on your mental health and wellbeing. Millions of people around the world wrestle with the socio-economic (and in some instances, political) changes that have taken place since the beginning of 2020.

How can it be that the desire for and an openness to change is so central to proactive behaviour, yet all indications (i.e. rising stress and mental health prevalence) suggest that we have a profound intolerance to uncertainty? Also, if "change" can create such high levels of distress for so many of us, how is it even possible to develop proactive behaviours as a resilience skill?

The answer to this conundrum is because most of us don't struggle with change in the broader sense, but rather we have an inability to respond to change. When change is imposed on us, it shakes us to the core. However, proactive behaviours differ in that they centre on initiating and driving the change. In many respects, change within this context takes place on our terms – we have control. This is the fundamental difference between being adaptable and proactive. Adaptability is a response to change, proactivity is the desire to create change.

There are three lessons in proactivity that can be drawn from Olympic champions:

Lesson 1
Actively look for opportunities in your life that will bring you fulfilment, purpose and happiness – don't settle for safety, complacency or comfort.

Lesson 2

When opportunities do finally emerge (with enough effort they eventually will), grab them and do your utmost to capitalise on every aspect of the journey.

Lesson 3

Bear in mind that the future you desire requires work and adaptability. Showing initiative, taking action and being persistent is central to transcending your environment and circumstances and achieving overall excellence.

SECTION SUMMARY

- Olympic champions have a broad repertoire of positive personality traits that support and promote resilience. These include extroversion, openness, conscientiousness, optimism, adaptive perfectionism and proactivity.
- Extroverts are able to draw energy from excitement, pressure and challenge.
- We all have the capacity to become extroverted within certain areas of our life should we choose to.
- Openness is a highly complex trait that brings imagination, feelings, ideas, values and aesthetics together with quickness, resourcefulness, competence, introspection and reflection.
- Openness is a primary measure of creative potential and achievements.
- Creativity is a predictive measure of resilience.
- Dopamine has the largest influence on creativity and openness.
- The environment we create for ourselves has a profound influence on dopamine production, transport and signalling.

- Dopamine can be increased and supported by cold immersion, aerobic exercise, enjoyable music, sunlight exposure, meditation and physical therapies.
- Conscientiousness is a significant resilience factor and happens to be one of the most impactful of all the positive personality influences.
- Conscientiousness includes being organised, planning ahead and being effective in goal setting and measured behaviours. It also encompasses a commitment to hard work, personal growth and achievement, which is augmented by self-discipline and self-control. Moreover, conscientiousness is associated with a greater degree of personal responsibility, accountability, reliability and high values.
- Proactivity is a trait that defines some of the world's top performers operating at the highest level.
- Adaptability is a response to change; proactivity is the desire to create change.
- Look for opportunities, show initiative and be persistent in your endeavours. When opportunites do finally present themselves, do not hesitate to grab them with both hands.

CHAMPION SKILL #4

MOTIVATION

Once something is a passion, the motivation is there.
MICHAEL SCHUMACHER

At the Tokyo Olympics in 2021, Dutch track star Sifan Hassan had a mission. Her mission was to successfully medal in three track-and-field events. This had only been achieved on two previous occasions in women's athletics, more than 70 years ago. Her chosen events included the 1,500, 5,000 and 10,000 metres. To compete in all three finals would require 24,500 metres of competitive track running over only nine days. To handle this kind of physical and mental load pushes the boundaries of human athletic performance. It is one thing to compete in both the 100- and 200-metre events, which take ±11–22 seconds respectively and are dominated by non-oxygen-dependent energy system contribution (anaerobic), but quite another to be competitive in the partially anaerobic 1,500 metres (±4 minutes) and another in the purely endurance-orientated 10,000 metres (±30 minutes).

On her first night, Hassan coasted to victory in the 5,000-metre qualifying event. She appeared to be on track and well prepared. However, three days later her dream almost came to an abrupt end in her 1,500-metre qualifying heat. Coming in to the final lap, Kenyan runner Edinah Jebitok tripped in front of Hassan, causing her to fall to the ground. With Hassan sprawled on the track, all seemed lost – certainly in the 1,500-metre event.

While most people would accept defeat based on uncontrollable external circumstances, Hassan motivated herself to get up. She exploded into an all-out sprint, with her sights fixed on the 12 elite competitors in front of her. Incredibly, she not only caught up, she passed all 12 competitors and went on to win the heat. From being flat on the ground, she ran those last 300 metres in 43 seconds.

Despite being in contention for the 1,500 metres, this all-out effort may have come at a price for Hassan. In less than 12 hours she was scheduled to compete in the 5,000-metre final event.

The adrenaline from the fall left Hassan wired – to the extent that she afterwards compared the experience to having drunk 20 cups of coffee. Personally, my limit is two cups a day, but I'm sure The Rock's energy drink will take you to that level pretty quickly!

According to Sifan: "I couldn't calm myself down, the whole day I was shaking. In the evening I was so tired."

As she warmed up for the 5,000-metre final later that evening, Hassan was sore all over (adrenaline is associated with increased muscle tension throughout the body as well as raised inflammation) and her doubts and lack of belief in herself became all-consuming. Yet, once she was in the race, she again found her spark, the motivation to dig deeper than ever before and won the event in 14 minutes and 36 seconds. Incredibly, despite the day's events, she was the 5,000-metre Olympic gold medallist – a childhood dream had come true.

But there was still work to be done.

Two days later, Hassan was back on the track and won her semi-final race in the 1,500 metres quite comfortably. By all accounts, she seemed to have fully recovered from her gruelling and challenge-filled week, or had she?

The 1,500-metre final did not go as Hassan had planned. Her strategy of pushing the pace too early backfired on her and she simply didn't have the energy reserves left and ended up receiving a bronze medal in a very respectable time of 3 minutes and 55.86 seconds. Despite her disappointment, with two events competed, Hassan had already been on the podium twice. Her final event was the 10,000 metres, which was scheduled to take place less than 24 hours later.

The week of competing had taken its toll and Hassan was physically and emotionally drained and in a great deal of pain. Moreover, the 10,000-metre event presented Hassan with a major barrier to winning gold, and that hurdle was in the form of the current world record holder in both the 5,000 metres and 10,000 metres and Hassan's arch-rival – Letesenbet Gidey from Ethiopia. Unlike Hassan, Gidey hadn't run five previous races by the time she lined up for the 10,000-metre event. She was fresh and had every intention of dominating the race. Over the years, the women's rivalry had become notoriously fierce, with many world records being broken in the process.

As expected, Gidey pushed the pace from the start and led for most of the race, but somehow Hassan was able to hang in. She waited patiently for the last turn of the last lap to strike – and strike she did. With 200 metres to go, she strode onto Gidey's shoulder and kicked for home. Hassan said she knew she'd won, but not much else registered.

"What happened just before and just after the finish line was a blur. Then, I wanted to celebrate," she said, "But when I finished I just fell down. I couldn't breathe."

When interviewed after the event, Hassan was asked what motivated or inspired her and how she managed to get up off the ground and go on to win the 1,500-metre qualifying race? How was she able to win gold later that day? These feats are seemingly impossible to the average person!

What many people don't know about Sifan Hassan's history is that in 2008 she arrived in the Netherlands on her own, in her early teens as an asylum seeker. For the first eight months, she lived at a refugee centre for minors in the north of Holland. Alone and scared, without anyone or anything familiar, she recalled crying herself to sleep every night. She was then moved to a home with other girls and it was there she disclosed her ambitions to one day become a runner. Shortly thereafter, Hassan was introduced to the Lionitas Athletics Club, where she met her first trainer, who lent her a 15-year-old pair of running shoes so that she could pursue her dream of running. It wasn't long before her talent was spotted and, as Hassan moved around Holland as part of her housing programme, she was introduced to better coaches and trainers. Always motivated and determined to be the best, she worked hard and grew into the star she is today.

Knowing her history, many people would have presumed that Hassan's response to what motivated her would be centred around never having to relive the pain of her past. Perhaps her success on the track would shield and buffer her from future hurt, vulnerability, insecurity and financial pressures. But to the surprise of those who were familiar with her painful past, Hassan's response to the question of motivation was such that it did not stem from fear, pain, rejection or punishment. Instead, her drive came from a positive set of emotions.

"For me, it is crucial to follow my heart," she said. "Doing that is far more important than gold medals. That keeps me motivated and it keeps me enjoying this beautiful sport."

Sifan loved to run – she was passionate about it. It brought her joy, a feeling of happiness, a sense of fulfilment and the experience of inner peace.

This joy, happiness and fulfilment is precisely what Fletcher and Sarkar found in their study of Olympic champions. Individually and collectively, they are incredibility motivated, to the extent that it is a significant resilience driver for them. What motivates Olympic champions is a deep passion for their sport or activity, achieving their predetermined goals and the recognition and sense of social value that is attached to their chosen path. At the same time, they are driven to be the best they can be in both their chosen sport and their lives.

■

FINDING THE BALANCE

Motivation (energised and persistent goal-directed behaviour) has been a topic of interest in research circles for many years. While the value of positive motivators has been clearly established in sports literature, there are other perspectives worth noting. There is also a fair amount of research supporting the notion that a focus on the possible negative outcomes related to a pursuit can also be a strong motivator and propel us with maximum velocity towards achieving our goals.

Imagine you are giving a high-level presentation for an exciting new business to a group of potential investors. What motivated you to create the business model in the first place may have been a passion for the industry, wanting to be the best at what you do, a love for your work and being able to capitalise on exciting market opportunities. However, when presenting your vision, every detail, the delivery and execution thereof is critically important in securing the necessary investor confidence and backing. For your goal to be realised (i.e. a well-funded and successful enterprise), the presentation/proposal requires hours of painstaking work, practice, repetition and exhaustive scenario modelling.

This begs the question as to what drives and motivates this arduous, but critically important process? Behavioural science shows us that by constantly recognising the implications and consequences of not being fully prepared for the presentation, which may include poor delivery, communication failure, overall disappointment and rejection, this realisation in itself acts as a powerful motivational force, nearly doubling our chances of success.

If we think back to Michael Phelps' psychological advantage and dominance over his rivals in competition, a lot of it had to do with the duality of his motivation. On the one hand, he would visualise the outcome he wanted for a race or event, driven by passion and a love for the sport. At the same time, he would role-play all the challenges that could arise and the consequences should he not prepare for any and every eventuality.

It appears that for the generation, maintenance and regulation of motivation, which are three sub-processes within the broader motivational context, a perfect mix of positive and negative drivers may be the way forward. However, while the negative motivators can support a desired outcome, the cost of ongoing fear, stress and hypervigilance must be taken into account. Chronically elevated stress responses due to catastrophising is ultimately antagonistic to resilience outcomes, not to mention overall health and wellbeing.

I have used both positive and negative motivators throughout my life. Coming from a childhood of neglect, abuse, relentless uncertainty and significant financial strain, my back was always against the wall and my footing insecure. Without a failsafe, I *had* to succeed in my endeavours, no matter the cost. Hypervigilance was a natural consequence of this perceived and lived reality and, as the years passed, the exhaustion and strain began to take a toll. Notwithstanding, I somehow still managed to achieve certain goals and lifelong aspirations. In my 40s, I underwent a fairly big shift when my core motivators became far more positive. Driven by a passion and love for what I do, striving to be the best that I can in my chosen endeavours and deriving significant meaning and purpose in my work, replaced the fear and anxiety about the possibility of failure.

This motivational shift has helped me to achieve a far greater flow in all that I have pursued since then. I have also found myself more absorbed in chosen experiences and challenges and have genuinely found joy and excitement in all my pastimes – most notably my work. There are many mornings when I enthusiastically jump out of bed at 4am, driven by the thrill and excitement of a current project or interest.

Taking both perspectives into account, combined with life experiences, I propose that the actual generation of motivation (which differs from the maintenance and regulation) for whatever we pursue in life should come from a positive place if it is to last.

Regardless of whether your motivation is positively or negatively driven, it is a complex behaviour involving around 15 brain structures, with the resilience powerhouse – the prefrontal cortex – at the epicentre.[1] Moreover, motivation is influenced and driven by the neurochemical dopamine.

> Dopamine is the primary driver of all forms of motivation.

In simple terms, what this means is that without a properly regulated and functional dopaminergic system, motivation (and ultimately resilience) will be difficult, if not impossible to achieve.

If you are someone who struggles to motivate yourself in certain areas of your life (i.e. getting up early, exercising, eating healthy food, etc.), it can be highly advantageous for your focus to be on promoting an optimal intrinsic environment for dopamine expression, and/or signalling and/or metabolism. By enhancing dopamine, you are able to experience greater motivation and drive, regardless of historical challenges in certain aspects of your life. Supporting dopamine is even more important if you have gene variants that are associated with a compromised dopaminergic system. The more influential genes include IL-6, DRD2, DRD4, DAT or COMT.

As mentioned, certain behaviours, such as aerobic exercise, cold immersion, meditation, sunlight exposure, massage and music, have a positive effect on dopamine, which is useful in the promotion of motivation. The table below provides a list of foods, beverages and nutrients that further augment dopamine expression and signalling.

Foods, nutrients and beverages that best support dopamine

Food, beverage or nutrient	Effects	Dosage or quantity	Considerations
Green tea	Improves/increases enzyme activity (tyrosine hydroxylase), which supports dopamine production. Green tea also slows the rate of dopamine reabsorption (through DAT inhibition), reduces the rate of dopamine metabolism (through the inhibition of monoamine oxidase B [MAO-B]), reduces damage to dopamine-producing cells (through increased antioxidant activity), reduces neuro-inflammation ($\downarrow$ IL-6), $\uparrow$ BDNF expression, which in turn supports dopamine.	**Tea:** 500–750 ml or 2–3 cups/day **Dosing:** Green tea extract (catechins) 100–800 mg/day **Ideal dosing:** 400 mg/day	Green tea is a great alternative to coffee for many reasons. Also, the caffeine content is a mere 25 mg as opposed to a brewed filter coffee, which contains as much as 63 mg.
Coffee	Increases sensitivity to dopamine and enhances its effects, i.e. signalling (due to upregulated D2 and D3 receptors).	**Healthy limits:** 2–3 cups/day **Caffeine upper limit:** 400 mg **Suggested timing:** Before lunchtime	Not everyone is able to consume coffee without adverse effects. Those with inherited polymorphisms in the CYP1A2 gene should limit coffee/caffeine. Additionally, those with gene variants that affect the stress axis should limit caffeine due to prolonged and/or exaggerated stress responses.

Food, beverage or nutrient	Effects	Dosage or quantity	Considerations
Tyrosine-rich foods	Tyrosine is a biological precursor and amino acid that is used to make dopamine. Ingestion of foods that are rich in this protein is associated with increased dopamine expression, which takes place within a period of 45–60 mins and can last from ±30 mins to as long as eight hours.	**Minimum daily requirements:** 1 gram/day **Ideal intake:** 1–2 grams/day **Best food sources:** Beef, fish, chicken, turkey, tofu, legumes (beans, lentils, chickpeas), pumpkin seeds, brown and wild rice, teff, oats, avocado	Tyrosine consumption is especially beneficial in situations where dopamine can become depleted, i.e. chronic stress and gruelling cognitive challenges. Studies reliably show that tyrosine improves cognitive and behavioural performance under adverse conditions, particularly when it is consumed prior to a challenge.
Omega-3 fatty acids	Can increase dopamine levels in the prefrontal cortex by up to 40% (possibly due to increased tyrosine hydroxylase expression). Omega-3 fatty acids are also associated with improved dopamine signalling, due to improved D2 receptor binding. Additionally, optimal levels of omega-3 fatty acids support and protect dopamine-producing cells (immune regulation) and slow the rate of dopamine breakdown (MAO-B inhibition).	**Dosing:** **Adult:** 1.5–2.5 grams/day **Adolescents (>9 years):** 1–1.6 grams/day **Children (<9 years):** 500–900 mg/day	Should you not wish to consume marine-derived omega-3 fatty acids (i.e. from salmon, herring, mackerel, krill, etc.) in supplemental form, consider regular consumption of the following foods: salmon, herring, sardines, mackerel, tuna, anchovies, sea bass, trout, snapper, sole, walnuts, chia seeds (high allergy warning), flax seeds, tofu, some beans, Brussels sprouts, avocado

Food, beverage or nutrient	Effects	Dosage or quantity	Considerations
Curcumin	The maximum effects of curcumin intake occur around 60 mins post ingestion. While higher doses do increase dopamine levels, the greatest benefit appears to be associated with reduced dopamine metabolism (inhibition of MAO-A and B). Curcumin also has powerful protective effects on dopamine-producing cells in the brain by dramatically reducing inflammation and oxidative stress.	**Dosing:** (Divided into three intakes) 1.5 grams/day (total amount) of curcumin + 6–7 mg/day piperine (absorption potentiator) or Meriva (curcumin + lecithin) 400 mg–1 gram/day Best taken with food	Curcumin is poorly absorbed and requires either fats or black pepper extract in order to address the issue.
Vitamin B9 (specifically methylfolate)	Methylfolate is central to the production of dopamine in that it supports and drives the enzymatic conversion of tyrosine into dopamine.	**Dosing:** (Taken once or twice) 400 mcg/day	Foods that are high in folate (vitamin B9) include: edamame beans, lentils, asparagus, spinach, broccoli, avocado, mango, lettuce, sweetcorn, oranges

MOTIVATION AND THE HABITS THAT SHAPE OUR FUTURE

In his book *Atomic Habits: Tiny Habits, Remarkable Results: An Easy and Proven Way to Build Good Habits and Break Bad Ones*, author James Clear describes a formula for creating successful habits that ultimately dictate our identity and reality.[2] One of the most striking statements that Clear makes in his book is: "Your identity emerges out of your habits. Every action is a vote for the type of person you wish to become."

Clear outlines a simple yet powerful formula for promoting positive change by creating new habits that involve creating a cue (a repeated experience), making it attractive, making it easy (to create frequency) and lastly to make the behaviour immediately satisfying. This four-step pattern is the foundation of every behaviour and habit we create in our lives.

The first stage of any new habit is a cue. The cue signals the brain to initiate a given behaviour as it's the piece of information that predicts an impending reward. For example, if I do this I can achieve success, receive praise, approval, love, friendship, satisfaction, admiration, etc. Creating an environment where there are constant reminders to behave in a certain way in order to achieve a desired outcome is a powerful first move.

The second part is making it attractive. This can be likened to the experience of a craving or, in more scientific terms, a dopamine spike. This in turn supports communication within the brain's reward centres. Here again, dopamine is a motivational force, as it underpins the deep appeal to positively shift one's internal state of being.

The third step is our response to perceived reward and a desire to change our internal state. This response depends on how motivated we are at the time (determined by levels of dopamine) and how much challenge/difficulty is associated with the intended behaviour. If the desired behaviour/task requires a lot of time, mental and/or physical energy, which we don't have or are not willing to expend, we simply won't do it – no matter the cue or perceived level of benefit. Therefore, matching the response to our abilities (the better we are in a given area, the easier a task is perceived), time and energy is vital.

For example, if we want to have greater clarity, focus and attention, there are many options that are available to us. One of the more effective habits would be to perform a full cold immersion in 8°C water for a period of 3–9 minutes. However, this process would probably require a trip to purchase 6–10 bags of ice, filling a bath, pouring the ice in and then finally a transient exposure to a very unpleasant and painful experience. The likelihood of someone who is not conditioned to the experience, or has not repeatedly felt the value and benefit of cold immersion by engaging in this habit, would be almost zero. Instead, drinking green tea or doing a short meditation would be a more practical and sustainable initial step. In simple terms, a new habit has to be easy.

The final aspect in the consolidation of a new habit is the reward. While we consciously consider the long-term implications of our behaviours, the appeal is the here and now and immediate contentment.

If you explore Clear's model within the framework of Olympic champions, it becomes apparent as to how and why they are able to maintain motivation and attain the performance heights that they do under some of the most difficult and challenging conditions imaginable.

The cues as an elite athlete are constant and the environment they live and train in very much supports their habits and journeys. They are up early, eat well and take nutritional supplements. Sport skill development and practice will dominate most mornings, while the afternoons belong to small skill refinements, physical development and loads of therapies. In many respects, it is a highly repetitive and subsequently an automated process, 365 days a year.

It is Clear's three other positive habit factors that are strongly influenced by the nature (i.e. positive or negative) of the motivation itself. When athletes are driven primarily by fear, pain, rejection and punishment (I have worked with many who are), it is very difficult for them to find that sense of attractiveness, ease and satisfaction within the self-development process, making the successful implementation of the necessary systems for goal realisation difficult to sustain, let alone master.

Unless we are constantly hacking our behaviours and "tricking" our system into positive habits (which is very attainable, as Clear points out, by following his process), repeated success in competition/life may be difficult to achieve, especially under more challenging and adverse conditions.

Conversely, when we are motivated by fire and passion, a love for what we do, joy and fulfilment, proficiency and goal realisation, the processes required to develop the mental, physical and emotional habits that culminate in resilience come more easily and naturally, are attractive and deeply satisfying.

Not only do positive motivators drive resilience behaviours, they drive something even greater – inspiration! It is only when we are inspired that we are able to pick ourselves up off the track, laden with disappointments and failures, pass our toughest competitors (which is often ourselves) and win the race of our life.

Michael Mankins, in his book *Time, Talent, Energy: Overcome Organisational Drag & Unleash Your Team's Productive Power*, describes the immense power of inspiration.[3] Although Mankins' context relates to businesses and organisational performance, in many ways these concepts and principles can be applied to our own lives in almost every context. Exhaustive research by Bain & Company (of which Mankins is a senior partner) has shown that contentment within your place of work (as opposed to being unhappy) will increase productivity by as much as 40 per cent. As a leader and/or manager of people, a happy environment can be created by reducing your team's stress (something I discuss in detail in my second book, *Stressproof: The Game Plan*), being more supportive, appreciative and providing opportunities for personal growth.

As remarkable as this increase in productivity is, it doesn't measure up to being fully engaged. Better engagement is augmented and supported by the feeling of a sense of personal control (a major contributor to motivation) and being accountable, feeling valued and important (yet another driver in intrinsic motivation), by growing and developing our skills and, most importantly, feeling that we are part of a supportive and unified team. This environment can increase individual productivity by 88 per cent when compared to an unhappy environment.

However, when we feel inspired, i.e. our motivation emanates from a place of passion, joy, fulfilment and where we are striving to be the best we can be and are free from self-imposed limitations, our productivity soars to a staggering 175 per cent above that of an unfulfilled life.

It is widely considered that self-discipline and constructive habits surpass motivation in the promotion of resilience and overall success. I subscribe to this and can relate to those behaviours wholeheartedly as they are central to my being. But the lesson that Olympic champions teach us is one where finding your deepest spark, together with your most authentic motivation, may actually precede self-control, self-discipline and positive habits.

To explore this on a personal level, ask yourself the following questions at least once a month:

- What motivates me to keep going when faced with challenges, obstacles, failures, traumas and setbacks?
- What motivates me to develop myself further, grow my skills and improve overall?
- What inspires me?

Drive checklist	My drivers (write a shortlist of three in each box)
What currently motivates me?	
What motivates me to develop myself further?	
What inspires me?	

The motivation analyses on p.221 will take some time to complete and will require some introspection. Once you have completed the questions, take a photo and print it out. That way, every time you experience a failure or setback or feel overwhelmed, read your answers out loud and re-centre your thoughts.

SECTION SUMMARY

- Olympic champions show exceptional motivation, even in adversity.
- Elite athletes are motivated by a passion for the sport, achieving goals, the recognition they receive from peers and by being the best they can be.
- Dopamine underpins and drives motivation.
- There are many genes that can influence dopamine expression, transport and signalling. These include IL-6, DRD2, DRD4, DAT and COMT. Gene testing can be extremely useful.
- In order to create a new habit, we require a cue and there needs to be a level of attractiveness, ease and satisfaction associated with the behaviour.
- When we are motivated by fear, pain, rejection and punishment, it becomes difficult to find ease, attractiveness and satisfaction in any new endeavour.
- When we are motivated by fire and passion, a love for what we do, joy and fulfilment, proficiency and goal realisation, the process required to develop the mental, physical and emotional habits that culminate in resilience come more easily, naturally and are attractive and deeply satisfying.
- Positive motivators are able to promote inspiration.
- The experience of happiness increases productivity by 40 per cent. Being fully engaged in an activity will increase productivity by 88 per cent. Being inspired (i.e. motivated by positive drivers) increases our productivity by 175 per cent.

CONFIDENCE

That was my way of getting through difficult times of low confidence – HARD WORK.

DAVID BECKHAM

Like the positive personality traits, such as extroversion, an openness to new experiences, conscientiousness, optimism, adaptive perfectionism and proactivity and motivation, self-confidence is very strongly associated with enhanced resilience and reduced vulnerability to adversity. Confidence can be described as the degree of certainty we have about our ability to be successful. This trait is fundamentally driven by successful outcomes in our chosen endeavours. The more successful we are in a particular area, the greater our confidence – right? You would think so, but self-confidence is considerably more complex than that. There is a fragility to this personality trait that transcends a history of repeated success.

BUILDING CONFIDENCE THROUGH ADVERSITY

Over the span of her 31-year professional career, my former client Martina Navratilova had won 59 Grand Slam titles (including nine Wimbledon titles), 167 singles titles, was voted Player of the Year on the WTA tour seven times and has been chosen as one of the Top 40 athletes of all time.

One of the highlights of my career was being part of Martina Navratilova's team in preparation for her final Grand Slam event – the 2006 US Open. I remember that two-week period vividly, largely due to the raised emotion surrounding her final matches and being part of tennis history, albeit in a small way.

Another contributing factor to the hype at the time was Maria Sharapova's (another former client who has shown exceptional resilience throughout the course of her career) dominance in the women's singles; her form had been sensational that year and both the media and fans soaked up every moment.

In the doubles, Martina was teamed up with Nadia Petrova, a powerful Russian player ranked number 3 in the world and who dominated the singles circuit at the time. In the mixed doubles, Navratilova's partner was one of the best doubles players of all time, the sensational Bob Brian.

One of my greatest memories of the event was the experience of the crowd's love and admiration for Navratilova. Every time she hit the ball, swung a racquet or spoke to her partner, fans cheered, applauded and went crazy. Echoes of "Come on, Martina", "We love you", "You're amazing, Martina" filled the stadium for the duration of all of her matches. She continues to be one of the most adored players of all time. She cares deeply about others and is involved in charities for animal rights, gay rights and underprivileged children. This, coupled with the fact that despite being ranked number 1 for 332 weeks, she is, and always has been, extremely humble.

With so much support behind her and a history of 167 singles titles, you would expect the tennis superstar to be brimming with confidence. But what would surprise many (including her opponents) is that this was in fact not the case. Before every match, Navratilova was very nervous, lacked self-confidence, experienced a significant degree of self-doubt – not dissimilar to the rest of us. Yet, she was about to secure another Grand Slam champion title in her final event, so it begs the question how or why did this overt lack of confidence not affect her final result?

Another iconic tennis player who has struggled with self-confidence throughout his career is Raphael Nadal, considered to be one of the greatest men's player in the history of the game, winning a total of 22 Grand Slam titles (Djokovic has won 23 and Federer 20) and spending 209 weeks as world number 1. Like Navratilova, his periodic lack of confidence is not reflected in his results.

What defines these two supreme athletes is that in those moments of self-doubt, low self-esteem and fear, they, like all successful Olympians, knew exactly what to do and how to respond. Fletcher and Sarkar found in their study of Olympic champions that they were able to derive confidence from several independent and outside sources, which included extensive and multifaceted preparation, visualisation, self-awareness and perceived esteem support from coaches and teammates.

The study also highlighted that the older, more experienced and more accomplished athletes (as was the case with Navratilova and Nadal) tended to struggle with confidence more than their younger counterparts. Yet, they did not experience a decline in performance as a result of this lack of self-belief.

The possible reason for this non-linear relationship between perceived confidence and performance outcomes was that Olympic gold medallists (Nadal also happens to be one) were able to bolster their confidence by drawing additional support off the people around them. The study proposed that coaches, trainers, psychologists, mentors, partners, family members and friends buffered the potential detrimental effects of a lack of confidence on sporting accomplishments. I have experienced this first hand with many athletes, on many occasions, including Martina and Maria, who just needed a subtle reminder as to how good they really were and how successful they had already been in situations like the one they were facing and, most importantly, the degree of preparation that had gone into the current event. You only need to watch a tennis match and count how many times some players look to their box for reinforcement and security to fully appreciate how influential support is within the confidence framework.

While this does explain a positive and critically important relationship that we can draw off in our own lives, it does not clarify the mechanism by which strong, authentic and meaningful relationships can promote self-confidence and increase our experience of self-worth. Understanding in this area could further serve to strengthen and enhance this influential resilience trait. My suspicion is that it has a lot to do with increased oxytocin expression and signalling and the neurochemical's profound role in stress responses and human behaviour.

■

OXYTOCIN, CONFIDENCE AND PERSONAL SUCCESS

There has been some insightful research in the area of high-level sports performance and the effects of oxytocin that may go some way to expand on this theory.

A 2010 study done at the University of Groningen in the Netherlands on professional soccer players looked to correlate celebratory behaviour and team support (known oxytocin triggers) with performance out-comes.[1] In other words, do winning teams celebrate more? Soccer is famous for its colourful characters, flamboyant victory moves and over-the-top team celebrations.

The research team focused on penalty shoot-outs and carefully analysed 325 penalties over a period of three decades in World Cup and European Championship matches. The study showed that the greater the celebratory behaviour by the player and/or the team, the higher the probability of them winning the match – the suspected driver being the increased expression of oxytocin.

In a team event, oxytocin's impact on outcomes can largely be attributed to its influence on those psychological behaviours that drive and contribute to group success. These include generosity, selflessness, cohesion, cooperation and motivation. However, the most striking effect of all is oxytocin's ability to promote and improve trust.[2] By trust, I am referring to the trust we have in our team, the trust we have for a process/journey and the trust we have in ourselves. Together with stress modulation, this is what oxytocin brings to the resilience experience.

Yet, there is still an additional advantage to oxytocin when experiencing adversity, challenge and struggle: it promotes highly predictive tendencies. This neuropeptide supports the recognition of the emotional states of others and enhances perceptual processes, including the ability to predict the way people are going to move and their future actions. In other words, oxytocin helps athletes more effectively and in real time to predict their opponents' level of focus, confidence, competitiveness and intended actions.

Imagine raising and supporting oxytocin's effects a day or two prior to delivering a critical live presentation. In this scenario, you are able to read the room and each person and their intended actions more accurately, which helps support your messaging, increasing the effectiveness of your pitch delivery. Or, consider running a workshop for your team where the body language and the facial expressions of others serve as rapid and clear cues for your tone, content direction and even necessary pauses.

The research suggests that by supporting oxytocin (probably over extended periods as opposed to sporadic intervals) this is the reality you can create.

Supporting this assertion, the following study was done in 2021 on young football players by a large team of Italian academics. What the researchers found was a direct correlation between oxytocin levels and sporting success.[3] The small study involved 56 players from different teams who were sampled (using a saliva swab) for oxytocin and cortisol

Activities that support and increase oxytocin

Activity	Outline	Required frequency
Prosocial behaviours	Connect more to the people in your life. Show them more support, care, compassion, empathy and give of yourself where possible.	Try to exceed more than 11 prosocial acts a week
Visceral manipulation	Visceral manipulation, sometimes referred to as visceral osteopathy, is fast becoming one of the most valued and sought-after practices within conservative healthcare. In my book *The Stress Code*, I explain many benefits and ways to locate a practitioner.	Once a week or twice a month for a period of 15–45 mins
Massage and physical therapies	Light to moderate pressure in the back and torso regions is able to achieve a 17% increase in oxytocin expression.	15 mins or longer, several times a week
Aerobic exercise	Running, swimming, hiking, cycling, tennis and soccer can increase oxytocin expression by as much as 250%.	15 mins or longer
Yoga	Consistent yoga practice over a period of a month can raise oxytocin levels by 450%.	15–45 mins several times a week
Slow relaxing music	Listening to relaxing music with a tempo of 60–80 beats a minute can increase oxytocin by 9.5% in a single session.	30 mins or longer

levels at two separate time intervals – 96 and 24 hours before a competitive match. The research team also measured their levels of anxiety and self-confidence using the Competitive State Anxiety Inventory-2 (CSAI-2). The CSAI-2 is a sport-specific, self-report questionnaire comprising 27 items pertaining to three subscales of anxiety (the fear of negative social evaluation, fear of failure and loss of self-esteem) and self-confidence (belief or degree of certainty that individuals possess about their ability to be successful in sport).

The results were astonishing and will most certainly spark further research into the performance-enhancing effects of oxytocin, because the study discovered that the winning teams had significantly higher oxytocin levels 24 hours prior to the match. They also showed lower cortisol and reported higher self-confidence and lower anxiety levels, suggesting that oxytocin may be predictive of results.

The table on p.228 shows specific activities that can increase the expression of oxytocin, confidence, resilience and performance and are a great complement to the oxytocin-boosting foods and nutrients listed in Part 2, Lesson 6.

If you have had a genetic test and uncovered polymorphisms in the OXTR gene, then, performed regularly, these activities can be helpful in reducing vulnerability to adversity, not to mention the optimisation of personal performance.

■

SECTION SUMMARY

- Self-confidence is positively associated with resilience.
- Confidence is the degree of certainty we have about our ability to be successful in a given endeavour.
- Olympic champions know how to respond to feelings of low confidence as a result of failures, disappointments and setbacks.
- Elite athletes derive their confidence from several independent sources, which include extensive preparation, visualisation, self-awareness (i.e. genetic profiling, blood work, fitness tests) and meaningful support from coaches and teammates.
- Oxytocin is the primary molecule that promotes feelings of self-confidence and self-esteem.
- Oxytocin drives team success by increasing generosity, selflessness, cohesion, cooperation, motivation and trust.
- Oxytocin supports the recognition of the emotional states of others and enhances perceptual processes, including the ability to predict the way people are going to move and future actions.

- Oxytocin brings stress reduction, predictive tendencies and increased trust to the resilience experience.
- Raised level of oxytocin prior to an event (24 hours) is associated with a considerably greater likelihood of success.
- By increasing oxytocin, one is able to increase self-confidence.
- Prosocial activities (care, empathy, charity, support, deep connection, encouragement), regular physical contact, visceral manipulation, physical therapies, aerobic exercise, yoga, slow relaxing music, taking quercetin, vitamin C, magnesium L-threonate, Lactobacillus reuteri and vitamin D can increase oxytocin.

FOCUS

Champions keep playing until they get it right.
BILLIE JEAN KING

Fletcher and Sarkar's study on Olympic champions also found focus to be an important feature of resilience in the athletes. This is hardly surprising if we consider Michael Jordan, Michael Phelps, Maria Sharapova, Serena Williams and Novak Djokovic, who all exude intense focus, both during practice and competition. It's the look in their eyes, their use of language during interviews and, if you have had the opportunity to meet them, it is very much in the way they carry themselves.

THE POWER OF TARGETED ATTENTION

Kevin Anderson was always passionate about tennis. As a boy, he and his family dreamed of him one day playing in the men's Wimbledon final – the sport's ultimate achievement. Anderson's aspirations to rise to the top of world tennis were well supported by a multitude of systems and processes, which included several hours of intense practice every day, eating the right foods, engaging in supplementary strength, speed, agility, flexibility and endurance training and, when warranted, physical therapies. This was his chosen life from the age of six or seven.

However, like many junior tennis players, Anderson was extremely prone to injury due to the endless hours on the court – 4–6 hours a day – the explosive and jarring nature of the sport and the relentless pressures from coaches and family. This was how we first met. Despite being only in his early to mid-teens, he was extraordinarily tall, having to bend down to walk through a standard doorway. In many respects, he resembled a basketball player more than a tennis player. It was little wonder that he struggled with injuries to the extent that he did. On our initial meeting, I really felt a connection to Kevin, his family, their values, struggles and their journey. My initial role was to help Kevin recover from his existing injuries as well as prevent future injuries and, in addition, assist in increasing his performance and overall potential.

In the early part of the 2000s, I was working with most of the top South African tennis players, largely due to my role as athletic director for the Davis Cup team. It was an exciting period, with training camps in the Western Cape and KwaZulu-Natal, the regular team-building exercises, flying to tournaments in interesting and remote countries and the overall passion and comradery that existed within the group of players and coaches. By extension, the squad was also trying to groom the next generation of players by including some of the more talented juniors.

But unfortunately for Kevin, he was just on the periphery of this group of talented junior players and therefore not included in the junior elite squad. While the coaches acknowledged that he showed promise, he was still developing and his process was less than orthodox (i.e. he had chosen to be parent-coached and managed) by South African standards and this unnerved many coaches and players. I became heavily invested in Kevin's success and tried to use some of my influence in the team to get the top juniors to practise with him and include him in their squad from time to time. To my disappointment, they refused and argued that he would bring their game down and they didn't have time to waste.

To be quite candid, it was infuriating. My frustration was that some of the team members were not taking the time or making the effort to explore the potential that existed beneath the surface. Kevin's effort, commitment, drive, passion and work ethic were simply unparalleled.

Fortunately, some of the senior players were more open to the idea and did include Kevin in some of the short training camps. Wesley Moodie, the 2005 Wimbledon doubles champion was a great support in this regard. Wesley had such a strong moral compass and was very gentle and caring. In all the years I worked with him, he always did what was right and not what was popular.

Remarkably, Kevin was able to disassociate from the exclusionary sentiment, judgement and hostility towards him and, despite experiencing hurt, rejection and isolation, he was able to channel the pain into further motivation and kept his focus on his journey and his process.

The one thing that really stood out about Kevin was that at the end of each day he would always reflect on what he had accomplished and what aspects of his game he had managed to improve upon. At the same time, he would ask key questions of himself and his team.

HOW I CAN DO BETTER TOMORROW? WHERE CAN I IMPROVE?

Remarkably, Kevin's focus was never on the external circumstances, which were largely beyond his or anyone's control. Instead, his singular attention was on his personal development, the process and journey, and he never allowed doubt to invade his thoughts or engaged in any form of distraction from his goals and aspirations.

As it turned out, when those senior players retired many years later, they were not replaced by the "groomed" juniors, leaving a gaping hole in South African representation on the professional circuit. In fact, none of the "new generation" players reached any measure of success in the professional game whatsoever. It was not through the lack of talent and ability but rather the dangerous combination of talent, arrogance and laziness.

Kevin leveraged off his intense focus and filled that void, exploding onto the circuit with incredible presence. Along with Kevin Curren back in 1985, Kevin Anderson became South Africa's top-ranked singles player in the history of the sport and reached a career high of number 5 in the world.

The dream of competing in the Wimbledon final finally did come true when he faced Novak Djokovic in the men's Wimbledon final in 2018. Unfortunately for Kevin, his semi-final victory over the tall American, John Isner, which lasted six hours and 36 minutes (the second longest match in the history of Wimbledon) had taken a physical toll on his health and affected his performance two days later in the final. Kevin received the runner's-up trophy that year.

Kevin had an incredible career, beating the likes of Roger Federer, Novak Djokovic (at the Miami Masters and Laver Cup) and Andy Murray. As Michael Phelps' coach, Bob Bowman, says, "dream big", and focus on your journey and the steps that you need to take to get you there.

Athletes don't have exclusivity in the area of focus. Each and every one of us has the ability to focus our attention, even those suffering with conditions where focus seems elusive, as is the case with ADHD.[1] The issue within the context of resilience and its relationship to focus relates more to the direction, target and regulation of our attention.

Our focus can be misguided and/or distilled as it was during the initial waves of the COVID-19 pandemic, when much of the world's attention was fixated on the uncertainties pertaining to the virus and its spread. While being informed was important in mitigating stress, in many instances the media hype became all-consuming, leaving many of us little to no time, energy or resources to focus on the necessary steps required to successfully navigate an uncertain future. In the same vein, some injured athletes incorrectly focus their attention on what the competition is doing, how they are training, how they are performing and where they are competing, to the extent that they partially neglect their own recovery and development.

What Kevin Anderson and the 12 Olympic champions can teach us is that focus is a primary resilience driver, but only when it is directed and controlled. So often in life we get drawn into events and circumstances that don't have any bearing on our experiences. If we want to adapt and thrive in new realities and amid volatility, it is important to remain *true to what we need to do* on our journey and, most importantly, the steps that are required to achieve this.

■

ZOOMING OUT

One additional learning in this area is a small piece of critical information pertaining to focus that was uncovered by Fletcher and Sarkar in their study. This insight pertains to the concept of unfocus.

When confronted with challenges, pressure, change, uncertainty, hardship and struggle, many of us (including myself) revert to a state of hypervigilance. In this state, we choose not to rest until a certain level of order and certainty is restored. The problem in this regard is that prolonged hypervigilance can lead to sleep disorders, fatigue, burnout, irritability and, in some cases, major anxiety. With few exceptions, we have all been thrust into a world of complexity and overwhelming uncertainty, affecting every aspect of our lives. An inability to take moments in the day or in the week to unfocus will eventually compromise resilience.

Where Olympic champions have a tremendous advantage is in their ability, learnt early in their athletic journey, to unfocus. Maria Sharapova managed to create unfocus opportunities in her career through a broad diversity in interests. She loved arts and culture and, during major events, she walked around the city, whether it was Melbourne, London or Paris, and explored the local stores, restaurants and galleries, speaking to curators, artists and restaurateurs about industry trends, life and everything in between. This gave her a different perspective, one outside of tennis and its pressures, expectations and demands. It provided her with a fresh lens, giving her that much-needed mental reset.

Personally, I am still working on the unfocus aspect and have a little way to go in this regard, but I fully understand and acknowledge its role in resilience.

SECTION SUMMARY

- The ability to focus is important in the promotion of resilience.
- We all have the ability to focus our attention, even those who are perceived to struggle in this regard.
- Olympic champions have an incredible ability to control the direction, regulation and target of their attention through adversity.
- Often during stressful events we focus on the wrong things and irrelevant content.
- Should we wish to adapt and thrive in new realities and amid volatility, it is important to focus on what we need to do, our journey and, importantly, the steps that are required to achieve this.
- Elite athletes create unfocus opportunities on a regular basis, especially during challenging periods. This encompasses activities that are completely unrelated to the primary demands, stress and challenges that exist at the time.

CHAMPION SKILL #7

SOCIAL SUPPORT

Be strong, be fearless, be beautiful. And believe that anything is possible when you have the right people to support you.

MISTY COPELAND

The importance of social support in resilience cannot be quantified. There is simply no equal. One of the greatest moments epitomising the power and value of social support culminated at the Tokyo 2021 Olympics when Italian high jumper, Gianmarco Tamberi, realised that he was an Olympic champion after an impeccable jump of 2.37 metres. The high-jump final took more than two-and-a-half hours to complete and is widely considered to be the most competitive in Olympic history. As the announcement was made, Tamberi leapt into the air repeatedly before collapsing face down on the ground. With his hands covering his face and tears streaming down both cheeks, Tamberi rolled back and forth. Eventually, he managed to stand up and then held his chest with both hands. This sequence of overwhelming emotion was repeated over and over again for the better part of two hours, which begs the question – why did he have such an emotional response (some may say disproportional) to victory?

I was deeply moved by Tamberi's joy and ecstasy, and his raw emotion was unmatched at the games that year, no mean feat considering many of the remarkable athletic accomplishments achieved. What made his accomplishment so extraordinary, and what explained his deeply moving reaction to winning the gold medal, was the road he had taken to get there.

Five years before the Tokyo Olympics, at the final event of the season with only 20 days to go before the Rio 2016 Olympics, Tamberi was in peak form. He had just jumped 2.39 metres and was attempting to enter the exclusive 2.40-metre club, which has only 11 members in the history of the sport.

Tamberi took a deep breath, his eyes focused intensely on the horizontal bar and launched into his run-up, gaining speed with every step. As he took his jump, something appeared to be off and on landing he grasped his foot with both hands. Immediately, he raised his arm calling for medical support. The stadium was silent and his coaching team were holding their breath. This couldn't be happening, not with Rio less than three weeks away.

Only when Tamberi slid off the mat and placed weight on his left foot did he and the rest of the stadium realise the magnitude of his injury. Tamberi fell to the ground and began to sob – in many respects not dissimilar to his 2021 Olympic victory celebrations, but on this occasion the tears were driven by agonising pain and shattered dreams. Tamberi was carried off the track on a stretcher, and later he had to have emergency surgery for a ruptured ligament and torn capsule. His Olympic journey, his life's purpose, his defining mission was potentially over for good.

Tamberi underwent intensive rehabilitation and, unbelievably, through hard work, discipline, persistence and determination, he was able to compete again in the 2017 season, despite medical opinions that said it may never be possible to jump again. But Tamberi's comeback was disastrous. In the second event of the year, the Diamond League meeting in Paris, Tamberi came in last, unable to clear his opening height. Having been at the summit of the sport, he was not even making an opening jump. According to Tamberi: "I was feeling a little like a baby competing with the adults. You know, sometimes there's a child that gets to play with adults and everyone tells them how good they are, they give them the ball and say 'Go, Go, Go'. That was me."

Following the event, Tamberi was inconsolable and locked himself in his hotel room and refused to come out or speak to anyone. Many of the organisers and athletes were deeply concerned for Tamberi's overall wellbeing.[1]

The next day, there was a forceful knock on his door. He repeatedly told the person to leave, but they refused. The knock became louder and more frequent and was accompanied by "GIMBO, GIMBO! Please I want to talk to you." Eventually, Tamberi conceded and let the person in.

"We talked. I cried in front of him. He tried to calm me down, and told me what he had to say," said Tamberi.

"Don't try to rush it," the person kept telling him. "You had a big injury, you're already back in the Diamond League. No one expected that. But now you need to take your time, don't expect too much too early from yourself. Just see what happens."

That moment was a turning point for Tamberi. Most people would assume that this person, who was able to lift Gianmarco when all hope appeared to be lost, was a parent, a coach, a sibling or even a partner – but it wasn't!

The person who made Tamberi believe in himself and his dream again was none other than Mutaz Barshim – his lifelong competitive rival.

The two went on to become inseparable and the closest of friends. In a "twist" of fate, one year later Barshim suffered the exact same injury and had to take a year off competing in order to recover. The day it happened, Tamberi spent the night in Mutaz's room, consoling him. Moreover, throughout Barshim's long and hard return to the sport, "Gimbo", as Barshim called him, encouraged him and lifted him whenever he felt lost and alone.[2]

The story doesn't end there. In Tokyo on that warm evening a few years later, Tamberi was not the only recipient of the gold medal in the men's high-jump event. For the first time since 1912, a joint gold was awarded and the other recipient was none other than Mutaz Barshim.

After the two athletes had completed their jumps, they were tied at 2.37 metres and, instead of a jump-off, the athletes asked officials if sharing the gold was an option. It was, and the rest is history. The motivation behind sharing the gold medal was not a fear of losing (they loved to compete) but rather not wanting to see their friend and training partner lose and experience disappointment.

Incredibly, it was through revealing their deepest vulnerabilities to each other that these rivals found their inner strength and ultimate success. Although their friendship came about in the most painful and difficult of times in both of their lives, at the Tokyo Olympics they had a once-in-a-lifetime opportunity to celebrate the best of times together – the joint realisation of dreams, with no losers, only champions, both on the track and in life.

According to Mutaz: "He's one of my best friends. Not only on the track but off the track. We're always together almost. This is a dream come true. It is the true spirit, the sportsman spirit, and we are here delivering this message."

He went on to say: "We have been through a lot, the same injury, and we know how much it takes, physically and mentally, just to get back here. I appreciate what he's done, he appreciates what I've done. This is amazing."

The Olympic motto of "Higher, Faster and Stronger" was rewritten in 2021 to include "Together", inspired by this historic moment.

Fletcher and Sakar's Olympics study found that the perception of social support from a variety of social agents underpinned the stress–resilience–performance relationship. In other words, Olympic champions know that without support they cannot be successful in managing their stress, and overcoming challenges, let alone achieving excellence. They, more than any other group, are aware that resilience is not partially but rather totally dependent on the support of others.

This is what made COVID-19 so difficult and unbearable for many of us. Being locked down, isolated and removed from friends, colleagues, teammates and family members at the very time that we needed each other the most, reduced individual resiliency on a global scale. There are those who may argue that phones, virtual platforms, social media and other means have sustained our connections and relationships, but most of us would agree that virtual communication does not have the same uplifting and supportive influence. This is because a large percentage of communication is non-verbal. Eye contact, touch, body language, facial expression and tone all contribute to our ability to connect and derive support from others.

Had Mutaz Barshim not been persistent and made his way into Tamberi's hotel room four years earlier and had Tamberi not opened up, exposing his fears, insecurities and emotional pain, this incredible result (two friends sharing the Olympic gold) would never have taken place.

We all have those moments when we pause to reflect on our successes and accomplishments. This may be related to work, sport, fitness-orientated, a creative achievement or something more personal. Often we will attribute our success to personal characteristics or environmental conditions, such as work ethic, passion, discipline, tenancy, ambition or even good timing. However, if you were to explore the circumstances that contributed to your accomplishments just a little deeper, and scratch just below the surface, you may be surprised to uncover that all the successes and achievements can be attributed to the support and guidance of others.

In my life's journey this could not be more true. While I have always had great ambition, worked really hard and been prepared to sacrifice much along the way, all my successes are because of others. There are people in my life who believed in me when I didn't believe in myself – who pushed me and forced me to grow when I was scared to move. There have been those who promoted me and encouraged me when I didn't feel worthy. And finally, from time to time, there have been a handful of people who have removed obstacles from my path. These people have been my teachers, friends, coaches, mentors and, of course, my exceptional wife, who has been the greatest of them all. My experience is not unique, it is a human condition and one that Olympic champions acknowledge and nurture.

TRUST AMPLIFIES THE VALUE OF SUPPORT

Although support is a central driver in resilience development and promotion, the Olympic study showed that for support to effectively reduce vulnerability to adversity, it needs to come from a source that is trusted and respected. In other words, trust forms the basis of social support and therefore resilience.

The *Oxford English Dictionary* offers the following definition of trust:

> *verb:* to have confidence in somebody; to believe that somebody is good, sincere, honest, etc.

Global communications firm Edelman is the world authority in the trust space. They partner with leading businesses and the world's top organisations to evolve, promote and protect their brands and reputations. Edelman has studied dynamic shifts in trust for more than 20 years and fully appreciate that trust defines an individual's, team's and organisation's licence to operate, lead and succeed. Trust is the ultimate currency, not only in the context of resilience but in all relationships.

According to Edelman, trust is based on two measures – competency (i.e. getting things done) and ethics (doing the right thing). What is intriguing is that trust is three times more dependent on ethics than competency.[3] What this means is that for support to properly translate to resilience, it needs to come from sources that are dependable, purpose-orientated and have the highest level of integrity. At the same time, we ourselves have to be receptive.

We have already discovered that the neurobiological basis for trust is the neuropeptide oxytocin, which suggests that should we wish to more successfully convert social support into personal resilience, it is important to promote stability within this system, especially in those with OXTR gene variants. For further details refer to Part 2 of this book.

SECTION SUMMARY

- Social support from a variety of social agents underpins the stress–resilience–performance relationship in Olympic champions and elite athletes.
- Many, if not all, of our greatest accomplishments and successes can be attributed to the contribution that others make to our lives.
- There is no substitute for human connection and care in the promotion of resilience, wellbeing and success.
- For support to promote resilience, it would have to come from a source that is trusted and respected.
- Trust forms the basis of social support and therefore resilience.
- Trust is the ultimate currency of all relationships.
- Trust is based on two measures: competency and ethics.
- For support to promote resilience it would need to come from a person and/or group that is dependable, purpose-orientated and lives their life with the highest levels of integrity.

DO YOU HAVE THE MINDSET OF A CHAMPION?

THE OLYMPIC GOLD TEST

The Olympic Gold Test assessment encapsulates the psychosocial and behavioural strengths of Olympic champions and high performers. It is based on several important resilience themes that can be compartmentalised into seven categories. Consider this test your "Future success playbook", providing you with the clarity to identify your current strengths and expose potential vulnerabilities.

How to interpret the assessment by category

Any section where you scored over 85 per cent should be considered a resilience/ superpower. These identified strengths will protect you in adversity and ensure success thereafter. They should not be neglected, but instead must be nurtured and continuously developed. It is also the area in which your contribution to the world around you is the greatest and the most magnified.

Conversely, should you score below 55 per cent in any category, it is suggestive of a current vulnerability. This area should be worked on in a slow, process-orientated way via the methods outlined throughout the book that cover these topics in great detail. For example, should you score low in the mindset category, in order to grow in this area you would need to strongly support the dopaminergic system through many of the activities contained within the book, including daily exercise, cold immersion, green tea, regular meditation and so on. At the same time, our challenges should be viewed not as a limitation but rather as a cue (if not an opportunity) to learn new skills, seek the advice of others (sometimes even if it's not what we want to hear) and double up on efforts.

Realise that this does take time, practice and repetition, so be kind to yourself when embarking on this, or any other resilience journey that requires new skills to be developed and old ones to be enhanced.

How to interpret the assessment overall

The assessment is out of a maximum score of 102 points.

Scoring

I have the mind of an Olympic champion: 85–102 points
I am en route to my personal Olympic gold: 70–84 points
I am resilient but have some work to do: 55–69 points
I am not there yet: 0–54 points

The Olympic Gold Test

Mindset	Yes, definitely (3 points)	Sometimes (2 points)	Seldom (1 point)	Never (0 points)
I see stress and challenges as personal growth opportunities				
Given enough time, I can learn and do almost anything I set my mind to				
I realise that success is determined by my efforts and attitude				
I am open to new experiences and willing to fail from time to time				
I value feedback from others, even if it's not always what I want to hear				
I find the success of others very motivating and inspiring				
SECTION SCORE				/18 points
Metacognition	Yes, definitely (3 points)	Sometimes (2 points)	Seldom (1 point)	Never (0 points)
When experiencing challenges and adversity do you use positive self-dialogue (i.e. I can do this one step at a time)?				
Do you still set and pursue short- and medium-term personal goals/aspirations even when confronted with long periods of stress and challenges?				
Do you practise visualisation (picturing all future realities, i.e. best case, worst case and most probable scenarios)?				
Are you able to recognise, control and regulate your stress responses?				
SECTION SCORE				/12 points

Positive personality	Yes, definitely (3 points)	Sometimes (2 points)	Seldom (1 point)	Never (0 points)
Are you outgoing and/or extroverted in any area of your life?				
Do you see possibilities that aren't always obvious to others?				
Do you try to understand the deeper meanings/concepts behind events?				
Do you strive to be well prepared and plan ahead?				
Are you committed to ongoing self-improvement and personal growth?				
In a difficult situation do you try to do the right thing?				
Would you describe yourself as good at reading events and situations, being open to change and action-orientated?				
Do you actively look for new opportunities in life?				
SECTION SCORE				**/24 points**
Motivation	Yes, definitely (3 points)	Sometimes (2 points)	Seldom (1 point)	Never (0 points)
In your work or primary pursuits are you intrinsically motivated by achieving goals, a passion for what you do and/or being the best at it?				
Are you able to stay motivated when facing adversity and challenges?				
Are you able to find inspiration in your daily life?				
SECTION SCORE				**/9 points**

Confidence	Yes, definitely (3 points)	Sometimes (2 points)	Seldom (1 point)	Never (0 points)
Are you able to remain intrinsically confident through successive failures and/or setbacks, even when you experience moments of self-doubt?				
When experiencing lower confidence, is your default response any of the following: intensify efforts and preparation, dive into self-exploration or recall past successes and achievements?				
Do you have strong social and emotional support structures?				
SECTION SCORE				/9 points
Focus	Yes, definitely (3 points)	Sometimes (2 points)	Seldom (1 point)	Never (0 points)
In stressful periods are you able to direct your focus constructively? (e.g. control where you direct your attention?)				
When experiencing difficulties are you able to disassociate from external events and what others are doing and saying?				
When stressed are you able to create unfocus opportunities where you take time in your day/week to engage in enjoyable activities?				
SECTION SCORE				/9 points

Social Support	Yes, definitely (3 points)	Sometimes (2 points)	Seldom (1 point)	Never (0 points)
Do you feel that you have good friends and strong emotional support structures?				
Do you feel that you have sound instrumental support (i.e. practical assistance) in your personal or professional life?				
Do you have people in your personal life who you trust and respect?				
Do you have people in your professional life who you trust and respect?				
Do others play a big role in your life?				
Do you perform aerobic exercise, meditation, yoga or charity work on a regular basis?				
Do you engage in regular therapies (physical or psychological) and/or take supplements like quercetin, vitamins D and C and magnesium?				
SECTION SCORE				/21 points
			Total score:	**/102 points**

CONCLUSION

Writing this book has been a very personal journey for me. I have had to relive both positive and negative experiences and reflect deeply on my life's journey up to this point. My wish is that there were (at the very least) moments when you as the reader were able to connect to a message, concept, theme, story or conversation in a meaningful and transformative way.

With few exceptions, we have all experienced some degree of struggle, hardship, failure, challenge, pain and sadness. For some it was in their formative years, while for others it was later in life. However, for most people the challenge is fairly constant, forcing us to draw heavily on emotional, mental and even physical resources day in and day out.

The conflict many of us are facing is that not only are we constantly expected to jump over hurdles, pull ourselves out of the trenches and get up after repeatedly being knocked down, we are also expected to find meaning and purpose in our lives along the way. For us to experience fulfilment, happiness and a sense of joy, we need to feel valued by others, that we are needed and even distinguish ourselves in those areas where our identity lies.

Resilience is the ultimate bridge between challenge and potential, potential and performance and performance and success. This is why *Thrive:*

A Practical Guide to Harness Your Resilience and Realize Your Potential is an ideal resource, providing the necessary skills for self-actualisation.

The first part of the book delivers the message of hope and transformation. Hope for a better future. Hope in that we are all endowed with exceptional gifts and abilities. Hope in the understanding that we have a unique mission in this world. Hope that our strongest fears and pervasive insecurities will eventually be replaced with self-confidence and higher purpose. Hope that even when all feels lost and we have no further to fall, our dreams can still be realised – because it's never too late.

The second section of the book looks at resilience through the lens of neuroscience. As the reader, you are plunged into the biological, genetic, behavioural and environmental drivers of resilience and human possibility. This set is complex, with many moving parts and layers and interdependent and interconnected relationships. By better understanding these factors, we are able to adopt the most opportune behaviours, relevant processes and ideal habits that will allow us to create the reality we want for ourselves, regardless of the circumstances we find ourselves in. Through extensive research, this section is also able to provide both objectivity and clarity that will help us to better make sense of our past experiences and traumas as well as contextualise current struggles. The combined effect of knowledge, understanding and actionable steps allows us to consciously choose our future path and ultimate destination in life.

The third part of the book gives us an extraordinary window into the mindsets, behaviours and attitudes that define many of the world's most accomplished and iconic athletes. Through this lens we are able to gain a behavioural science perspective in resilience realisation. I personally stepped into this extraordinary world in 2001. My intention was to enhance the careers and performance of these exceptional and talented individuals by making them faster, stronger, more powerful and injury resistant. Incredibly, my professional life has turned out to be a 20-year masterclass in human resilience. Through this journey, I was able to transform myself, leaving behind many of the psychological and emotional restraints of my past and stepped into the future with the knowledge that "I've got this'. It may seem abstract for us to draw lessons and inspiration from people who in many respects defy the limits of human capabilities. Yet, in truth, they are no different to us and they share the same struggles, values and goals. Their story is fundamentally our story and what sets them apart is a collective of acquired skills that are constantly refined and added to throughout the course of their lives.

We live in a time of great complexity, uncertainty and overwhelming vulnerability. Living in a constant state of hypervigilance, worry, fear, anxiety, frustration and sense of personal failure is not something we have chosen, instead it has been thrust upon us by several converging and interposed factors, which include the aftermath of COVID-19, the devastating war in the Ukraine and the socio-economic changes brought on by the 4IR.

While we have not consciously chosen a life of challenges and adversity, professional athletes are one of only two groups (the other being elite military units) who have. They have intentionally and purposefully opted for a life that is fraught with hardship, repeated failure, ongoing setbacks and constant disappointments.

They choose this path because, as hard as it may be, it offers opportunities for exceptional personal growth and development, unimaginable joy, unrestrained passion, excitement and the realisation of one's fullest potential – the ultimate prize. For elite athletes, the benefits far outshine the possible disadvantages and obstacles that need to be conquered. To be successful in their chosen path, elite athletes have to learn many resilience skills from a young age and at a level that most people would find far too daunting. Like their sporting ability, these skills ultimately differentiate them on the field, mat, court, ice, slopes and in life in general.

The skills that athletes require and foster are things that are as vital as those needed for high performers, such as executives, bankers, lawyers, doctors, artists, scholars, musicians, developers and engineers. They are no different to Olympic champions in that they too have made the decision to increase their exposure to stress, adversity, complexity and repeated setbacks. These resilience skills are pervasive in every sphere of life and link seemingly disconnected worlds.

Sporting champions are some of the finest examples of human resilience and are therefore the best teachers to guide us through the landscape we find ourselves in at this moment in history. They are a group of people who have, in a literal physical and mental sense, been training for stress and adversity their entire lives.

Beyond the many stories, lessons and self-explorations in this third and last section, we also learn that with deliberate effort we can more effectively leverage off our existing strengths. At the same time we are able to control the way we think, feel and act in any given situation – the choice is ours, it has always been. Moreover, we all have the potential to build our perceived weaknesses and greatest vulnerabilities into tactical weapons that will help us overcome almost any challenge and attain the goals we set for ourselves throughout life.

Together, the three parts converge to provide a powerful resilience framework, in many respects a playbook, that can be used to support us in the terrifying moments when we question ourselves, our value and our worth, and in periods when we want to exceed our own expectations.

In many respects, the life we live can be viewed as our own personal Olympics. We all have hopes and aspirations, we work hard, we commit ourselves and, for the most part, we achieve some measure of success. At the same time, we frequently fall, let ourselves and others down, and experience heartache and deep disappointment.

Yet, it is through both the successes and failures that we give ourselves the opportunity to stand on life's podium, holding our unique and deeply personal "gold medal". For dreams to become a reality, we can draw from those who have inspired us for well over a century – Olympians! Let us commit ourselves to adapting FASTER, rising HIGHER, becoming mentally and physically STRONGER and, finally, let us come TOGETHER. In this way, the only problem with a dream is the fact that it may not be big enough.

NOTES AND REFERENCES

Part 1: Understanding our potential

The ultimate story of resilience

1 https://www.cdc.gov/ncbddd/actearly/milestones/milestones-3yr.html
2 Criscuolo, Antonio, et al. "On the association between musical training, intelligence and executive functions in adulthood". *Frontiers in Psychology* 10 (2019): 1704.
3 Isaacson, Walter. *Einstein: His Life and Universe.* Simon & Schuster, 2007.
4 Grant, Adam. *Originals: How Non-conformists Move the World.* Penguin, 2017.
5 Galatzer-Levy, Isaac R., Sandy H. Huang, and George A. Bonanno. "Trajectories of resilience and dysfunction following potential trauma: A review and statistical evaluation". *Clinical Psychology Review* 63 (2018): 41–55.
6 Sutton, Richard. *Stressproof: The Game Plan.* Pan Macmillan, 2021.
7 Mestre, José M., et al. "Emotion regulation ability and resilience in a sample of adolescents from a suburban area". *Frontiers in Psychology* 8 (2017): 1980.

Part 2: The neuroscience of resilience

1 Malhi, Gin S., et al. "Modelling resilience in adolescence and adversity: A novel framework to inform research and practice". *Translational Psychiatry* 9.1 (2019): 1–16.

Lesson 1 : Personality

1 Oshio, Atsushi, et al. "Resilience and Big Five personality traits: A meta-analysis". *Personality and Individual Differences* 127 (2018): 54–60.

2 Ho, B.-C., et al. "Catechol-o-methyl transferase Val158Met gene polymorphism in schizophrenia: Working memory, frontal lobe MRI morphology and frontal cerebral blood flow". *Molecular Psychiatry* 10.3 (2005): 287–298.

3 Bozek, Tomislav, et al. "The influence of dopamine-beta-hydroxylase and catechol o-methyltransferase gene polymorphism on the efficacy of insulin detemir therapy in patients with type 2 diabetes mellitus". *Diabetology & Metabolic Syndrome* 9.1 (2017): 1–11.

4 Darbre, Philippa D. "The history of endocrine-disrupting chemicals". *Current Opinion in Endocrine and Metabolic Research* 7 (2019): 26–33.

5 Sagone, Elisabetta, and Maria Elvira De Caroli. "Positive personality as a predictor of high resilience in adolescence". *Journal of Psychology and Behavioral Science* 3.2 (2015): 45–53.

6 Latsko, Maeson S., et al. "A novel interaction between tryptophan hydroxylase 2 (TPH2) gene polymorphism (rs4570625) and BDNF Val66Met predicts a high-risk emotional phenotype in healthy subjects". *PLoS One* 11.10 (2016): e0162585.

7 Belsky, Jay, and Sarah Hartman. "Gene-environment interaction in evolutionary perspective: Differential susceptibility to environmental influences". *World Psychiatry* 13.1 (2014): 87.

8 Lesch, Klaus-Peter, et al. "Association of anxiety-related traits with a polymorphism in the serotonin transporter gene regulatory region". *Science* 274.5292 (1996): 1527–1531.

9 Ptáček, Radek, Hana Kuželová, and George B. Stefano. "Dopamine D4 receptor gene DRD4 and its association with psychiatric disorders". *Medical Science Monitor: International Medical Journal of Experimental and Clinical Research* 17.9 (2011): RA215.

10 Belsky, Jay, and Michael Pluess. "Beyond risk, resilience, and dysregulation: Phenotypic plasticity and human development". *Development and Psychopathology* 25.4pt2 (2013): 1243–1261.

Lesson 2 : Childhood

1 Green, Jennifer Greif, et al. "Childhood adversities and adult psychiatric disorders in the national comorbidity survey replication I: Associations with first onset of DSM-IV disorders". *Archives of General Psychiatry* 67.2 (2010): 113–123.

2 Kidman, Rachel, Luciane R. Piccolo, and Hans-Peter Kohler. "Adverse childhood experiences: Prevalence and association with adolescent health in Malawi". *American Journal of Preventive Medicine* 58.2 (2020): 285–293.

3 Soares, Ana Luiza Gonçalves, et al. "Adverse childhood experiences: Prevalence and related factors in adolescents of a Brazilian birth cohort". *Child Abuse & Neglect* 51 (2016): 21–30.

4 Stambaugh, Leyla F., et al. "Prevalence of serious mental illness among parents in the United States: Results from the National Survey of Drug Use and Health, 2008–2014". *Annals of Epidemiology* 27.3 (2017): 222–224.

5 McLaughlin, Katie A., et al. "Mechanisms linking childhood trauma exposure and psychopathology: A transdiagnostic model of risk and resilience". *BMC Medicine* 18.1 (2020): 1–11.

6 Chen, Edith, et al. "Association of reports of childhood abuse and all-cause mortality rates in women". *JAMA Psychiatry* 73.9 (2016): 920–927.

7 Kessler, Ronald C., et al. "Childhood adversities and adult psychopathology in the WHO World Mental Health Surveys". *British Journal of Psychiatry* 197.5 (2010): 378–385.

8 Kuhlman, Kate Ryan, et al. "Developmental psychoneuroendocrine and psychoneuroimmune pathways from childhood adversity to disease". *Neuroscience and Biobehavioral Reviews* 80 (2017): 166–184.

9 Sutton, Richard. *Stressproof: The Game Plan.* Pan Macmillan, 2021.

10 Sutton, Richard. *The Stress Code: From Surviving to Thriving.* Pan Macmillan, 2018.

Lesson 3: New challenges, new skills

1 https://www.gallup.com/workplace/349484/state-of-the-global-workplace.aspx

Lesson 4 : Resilience in the brain

1 Bolsinger, Julia, et al. "Neuroimaging correlates of resilience to traumatic events: A comprehensive review". *Frontiers in Psychiatry* 9 (2018): 693.

2 Nave, Gideon, et al. "Are bigger brains smarter? Evidence from a large-scale preregistered study". *Psychological Science* 30.1 (2019): 43–54.

3 Ansell, Emily B., et al. "Cumulative adversity and smaller gray matter volume in medial prefrontal, anterior cingulate, and insula regions". *Biological Psychiatry* 72.1 (2012): 57–64.

4 Chetty, Sundari, et al. "Stress and glucocorticoids promote oligodendrogenesis in the adult hippocampus". *Molecular Psychiatry* 19.12 (2014): 1275.

5 Stark, Ken D., et al. "Global survey of the omega-3 fatty acids, docosahexaenoic acid and eicosapentaenoic acid in the blood stream of healthy adults". *Progress in Lipid Research* 63 (2016): 132–152.

6 Delarue, J.O.C.P., et al. "Fish oil prevents the adrenal activation elicited by mental stress in healthy men". *Diabetes & Metabolism* 29.3 (2003): 289–295.

7 Pusceddu, M.M., et al. "The omega-3 polyunsaturated fatty acid docosahexaenoic acid (DHA) reverses corticosterone-induced changes in cortical neurons". *International Journal of Neuropsychopharmacology* 19.6 (2016): pyv130.

8 Witte, V.A., et al. "Long-chain omega-3 fatty acids improve brain function and structure in older adults". *Cerebral Cortex* (2013): bht163.

9 Wu, Aiguo, Zhe Ying, and Fernando Gomez-Pinilla. "Docosahexaenoic acid dietary supplementation enhances the effects of exercise on synaptic plasticity and cognition". *Neuroscience* 155.3 (2008): 751–759.

10 EFSA Panel on Dietetic Products, Nutrition and Allergies (NDA). "Scientific opinion on the tolerable upper intake level of eicosapentaenoic acid (EPA), docosahexaenoic acid (DHA) and docosapentaenoic acid (DPA)". *EFSA Journal* 10.7 (2012): 2815.

11 https://ods.od.nih.gov/factsheets/Omega3FattyAcids-HealthProfessional/#en30

12 Lane, Katie, et al. "Bioavailability and potential uses of vegetarian sources of omega-3 fatty acids: A review of the literature". *Critical Reviews in Food Science and Nutrition* 54.5 (2014): 572–579.

13 Ginty, Annie T., and Sarah M. Conklin. "Short-term supplementation of acute long-chain omega-3 polyunsaturated fatty acids may alter depression

status and decrease symptomology among young adults with depression: A preliminary randomized and placebo controlled trial". *Psychiatry Research* 229.1–2 (2015): 485–489.

14 Kiecolt-Glaser, Janice K., et al. "Omega-3 supplementation lowers inflammation and anxiety in medical students: A randomized controlled trial". *Brain, Behavior, and Immunity* 25.8 (2011): 1725–1734.

15 Fox, Kieran C.R., et al. "Is meditation associated with altered brain structure? A systematic review and meta-analysis of morphometric neuroimaging in meditation practitioners". *Neuroscience & Biobehavioral Reviews* 43 (2014): 48–73.

16 Dodich, Alessandra, et al. "Short-term Sahaja Yoga meditation training modulates brain structure and spontaneous activity in the executive control network". *Brain and Behavior* 9.1 (2019): e01159.

17 Tang, Yi-Yuan, et al. "Brief mental training reorganizes large-scale brain networks". *Frontiers in Systems Neuroscience* 11 (2017): 6.

18 Lutz, Antoine, et al. "Attention regulation and monitoring in meditation". *Trends in Cognitive Sciences* 12.4 (2008): 163–169.

19 Bellosta-Batalla, Miguel, et al. "Increased salivary oxytocin and empathy in students of clinical and health psychology after a mindfulness and compassion-based intervention". *Mindfulness* (2020): 1–12.

20 Fox, K.C.R., et al. "Functional neuroanatomy of meditation: A review and meta-analysis of 78 functional neuroimaging investigations". *Neuroscience & Biobehavioral Reviews* 65 (2016): 208–228.

21 Black, D.S., et al. "Yogic meditation reverses NF-κB and IRF-related transcriptome dynamics in leukocytes of family dementia caregivers in a randomized controlled trial". *Psychoneuroendocrinology* 38.3 (2013): 348–355.

22 Basso, Julia C., et al. "Brief, daily meditation enhances attention, memory, mood, and emotional regulation in non-experienced meditators". *Behavioural Brain Research* 356 (2019): 208–220.

Lesson 5: Intellect

1 Aldao, Amelia, Susan Nolen-Hoeksema, and Susanne Schweizer. "Emotion-regulation strategies across psychopathology: A meta-analytic review". *Clinical Psychology Review* 30.2 (2010): 217–237.

2 Grenell, Amanda, et al. "Individual differences in the effectiveness of self-distancing for young children's emotion regulation". *British Journal of Developmental Psychology* 37.1 (2019): 84–100.

3 Nook, Erik C., Jessica L. Schleider, and Leah H. Somerville. "A linguistic signature of psychological distancing in emotion regulation". *Journal of Experimental Psychology: General* 146.3 (2017): 337.

4 Tartar, Jaime L., et al. "The 'warrior' COMT Val/Met genotype occurs in greater frequencies in mixed martial arts fighters relative to controls". *Journal of Sports Science & Medicine* 19.1 (2020): 38.

5 Keers, Robert, and Katherine J. Aitchison. "Pharmacogenetics of antidepressant response". *Expert Review of Neurotherapeutics* 11.1 (2011): 101–125.

6 Crum, Alia J., et al. "Catechol-o-methyltransferase moderates effect of stress mindset on affect and cognition". *PLoS One* 13.4 (2018): e0195883.

7 Maul, Stephan, et al. "Genetics of resilience: Implications from genome-wide association studies and candidate genes of the stress response system in posttraumatic stress disorder and depression". *American Journal of Medical Genetics Part B: Neuropsychiatric Genetics* 183.2 (2020): 77–94.

8 Carneiro, Lara SF, et al. "Impact of physical exercise on catechol-o-methyltransferase activity in depressive patients: A preliminary communication". *Journal of Affective Disorders* 193 (2016): 117–122.

9 Dethe, Shekhar, M. Deepak, and Amit Agarwal. "Elucidation of molecular mechanism(s) of cognition enhancing activity of Bacomind®: A standardized extract of Bacopa monnieri". *Pharmacognosy Magazine* 12.Suppl 4 (2016): S482.

10 https://examine.com/supplements/bacopa-monnieri/#how-to-take

Lesson 6 : Support and connection

1 Dube, Shanta R., et al. "Cumulative childhood stress and autoimmune diseases in adults". *Psychosomatic Medicine* 71.2 (2009): 243.

2 Thomas, C., E. Hyppönen, and C. Power. (2008). "Obesity and type 2 diabetes risk in midadult life: The role of childhood adversity". *Pediatrics*, 121, e1240–e1249.

3 Slopen, Natalie, Karestan C. Koenen, and Laura D. Kubzansky. "Childhood adversity and immune and inflammatory biomarkers associated with cardiovascular risk in youth: A systematic review". *Brain, Behavior, and Immunity* 26.2 (2012): 239–250.

4 Ridout, Kathryn K., et al. "Early life adversity and telomere length: A meta-analysis". *Molecular Psychiatry* 23.4 (2018): 858–871.

5 Green, Jennifer Greif, et al. "Childhood adversities and adult psychiatric disorders in the national comorbidity survey replication I: Associations with first onset of DSM-IV disorders". *Archives of General Psychiatry* 67.2 (2010): 113–123.

6 Gunnar, Megan R., and Camelia E. Hostinar. "The social buffering of the hypothalamic–pituitary–adrenocortical axis in humans: Developmental and experiential determinants". *Social Neuroscience* 10.5 (2015): 479–488.

7 Hostinar, Camelia E., and Megan R. Gunnar. "Social support can buffer against stress and shape brain activity". *AJOB Neuroscience* 6.3 (2015): 34–42.

8 https://www.ipsos.com/en/loneliness-increase-worldwide-increase-local-community-support

9 Surkalim, Daniel L., et al. "The prevalence of loneliness across 113 countries: Systematic review and meta-analysis". *BMJ* 376 (2022).

10 Brown, Kirk Warren, Netta Weinstein, and J. David Creswell. "Trait mindfulness modulates neuroendocrine and affective responses to social evaluative threat". *Psychoneuroendocrinology* 37.12 (2012): 2037–2041.

11 Creswell, J. David, and Emily K. Lindsay. "How does mindfulness training affect health? A mindfulness stress buffering account". *Current Directions in Psychological Science* 23.6 (2014): 401–407.

12 Taren, Adrienne A., J. David Creswell, and Peter J. Gianaros. "Dispositional mindfulness co-varies with smaller amygdala and caudate volumes in community adults". *PLoS One* 8.5 (2013): e64574.

13 Carter, C. Sue, et al. "Is oxytocin 'nature's medicine'?" *Pharmacological Reviews* 72.4 (2020): 829–861.

14 Quintana, Daniel S., and Adam J. Guastella. "An allostatic theory of oxytocin". *Trends in Cognitive Sciences* 24.7 (2020): 515–528.

15 Sobota, Rosanna, et al. "Oxytocin reduces amygdala activity, increases social interactions, and reduces anxiety-like behavior irrespective of NMDAR antagonism". *Behavioral Neuroscience* 129.4 (2015): 389.

16 Linnen, Anne-Marie, et al. "Intranasal oxytocin and salivary cortisol concentrations during social rejection in university students". *Stress* 15.4 (2012): 393–402.

17 Kemp, Andrew H., et al. "Oxytocin increases heart rate variability in humans at rest: Implications for social approach-related motivation and capacity for social engagement". *PLoS One* 7.8 (2012): e44014.

18 Kirsch, Peter, et al. "Oxytocin modulates neural circuitry for social cognition and fear in humans". *Journal of Neuroscience* 25.49 (2005): 11489–11493.

19 Sripada, Chandra Sekhar, et al. "Oxytocin enhances resting-state connectivity between amygdala and medial frontal cortex". *International Journal of Neuropsychopharmacology* 16.2 (2013): 255–260.

20 Tarko, Adam, et al. "Effects of benzene, quercetin, and their combination on porcine ovarian cell proliferation, apoptosis, and hormone release". *Archives Animal Breeding* 62.1 (2019): 345–351.

21 https://examine.com/supplements/quercetin/

22 Kaviani, Mina, et al. "Effects of vitamin D supplementation on depression and some involved neurotransmitters". *Journal of Affective Disorders* 269 (2020): 28–35.

23 https://examine.com/supplements/vitamin-d/

24 Poutahidis, Theofilos, et al. "Microbial symbionts accelerate wound healing via the neuropeptide hormone oxytocin". *PLoS One* 8.10 (2013): e78898.

25 https:/examine.com/supplements/lactobacillus-reuteri/

Lesson 7: The immune system

1 Kim, Yong-Ku, and Eunsoo Won. "The influence of stress on neuroinflammation and alterations in brain structure and function in major depressive disorder". *Behavioural Brain Research* 329 (2017): 6–11.

2 Menard, Caroline, et al. "Social stress induces neurovascular pathology promoting depression". *Nature Neuroscience* 20.12 (2017): 1752–1760.

3 Troubat, Romain, et al. "Neuroinflammation and depression: A review". *European Journal of Neuroscience* 53.1 (2021): 151–171.

4 Strasser, Barbara, et al. "Mechanisms of inflammation-associated depression: Immune influences on tryptophan and phenylalanine metabolisms". *Inflammation-Associated Depression: Evidence, Mechanisms and Implications* (2016): 95–115.

5 Howard, Emily E., et al. "Divergent roles of inflammation in skeletal muscle recovery from injury". *Frontiers in Physiology* 11 (2020): 87.

6 Dantzer, Robert, et al. "From inflammation to sickness and depression: When the immune system subjugates the brain". *Nature Reviews Neuroscience* 9.1 (2008): 46–56.

7 Beurel, Eléonore, Marisa Toups, and Charles B. Nemeroff. "The bidirectional relationship of depression and inflammation: Double trouble". *Neuron* 107.2 (2020): 234–256.

8 Passos, Ives Cavalcante, et al. "Inflammatory markers in post-traumatic stress disorder: A systematic review, meta-analysis, and meta-regression". *The Lancet Psychiatry* 2.11 (2015): 1002–1012.

9 https://www.mayoclinic.org/diseases-conditions/post-traumatic-stress-disorder/symptoms-causes/syc-20355967

10 Michopoulos, Vasiliki, et al. "Inflammation in fear- and anxiety-based disorders: PTSD, GAD, and beyond". *Neuropsychopharmacology* 42.1 (2017): 254–270.

11 Imai, Risa, et al. "Relationships of blood proinflammatory markers with psychological resilience and quality of life in civilian women with posttraumatic stress disorder". *Scientific Reports* 9.1 (2019): 1–10.

12 Imai, Risa, et al. "Relationships of blood proinflammatory markers with psychological resilience and quality of life in civilian women with posttraumatic stress disorder". *Scientific Reports* 9.1 (2019): 1–10.

13 Schetter, Christine Dunkel, and Christyn Dolbier. "Resilience in the context of chronic stress and health in adults". *Social and Personality Psychology Compass* 5.9 (2011): 634–652.

14 Elliot, Ari J., et al. "Associations of lifetime trauma and chronic stress with C-reactive protein in adults ages 50 years and older: Examining the moderating role of perceived control". *Psychosomatic Medicine* 79.6 (2017): 622–630.

15 Veenhoven, Ruut. "Healthy happiness: Effects of happiness on physical health and the consequences for preventive health care". *Journal of Happiness Studies* 9.3 (2008): 449–469.

16 Pressman, Sarah D., Matthew W. Gallagher, and Shane J. Lopez. "Is the emotion-health connection a 'first-world problem'?" *Psychological Science* 24.4 (2013): 544–549.

17 Dantzer, Robert, et al. "Resilience and immunity". *Brain, Behavior, and Immunity* 74 (2018): 28–42.

18 Roy, Brita, et al. "Association of optimism and pessimism with inflammation and hemostasis in the Multi-Ethnic Study of Atherosclerosis (MESA)". *Psychosomatic Medicine* 72.2 (2010): 134.

19 Giltay, Erik J., et al. "Lifestyle and dietary correlates of dispositional optimism in men: The Zutphen Elderly Study". *Journal of Psychosomatic Research* 63.5 (2007): 483–490.

20 Rozanski, Alan, and Laura D. Kubzansky. "Psychologic functioning and physical health: A paradigm of flexibility". *Psychosomatic Medicine* 67 (2005): S47–S53.

21 Saphire-Bernstein, Shimon, et al. "Oxytocin receptor gene (OXTR) is related to psychological resources". *Proceedings of the National Academy of Sciences* 108.37 (2011): 15118–15122.

Lesson 8 : Health behaviours

1 Bell, Steven, et al. "Ten-year alcohol consumption typologies and trajectories of C-reactive protein, interleukin-6 and interleukin-1 receptor antagonist over the following 12 years: A prospective cohort study". *Journal of Internal Medicine* 281.1 (2017): 75–85.

2 Irwin, Michael R., et al. "Sleep deprivation and activation of morning levels of cellular and genomic markers of inflammation". *Archives of Internal Medicine* 166.16 (2006): 1756–1762.

3 Goletzke, Janina, et al. "Increased intake of carbohydrates from sources with a higher glycemic index and lower consumption of whole grains during puberty are prospectively associated with higher IL-6 concentrations in younger adulthood among healthy individuals". *Journal of Nutrition* 144.10 (2014): 1586–1593.

4 Kelly, Karen R., et al. "A low-glycemic index diet and exercise intervention reduces TNF-α in isolated mononuclear cells of older, obese adults". *Journal of Nutrition* 141.6 (2011): 1089–1094.

5 Kastelein, Tegan, Rob Duffield, and Frank Marino. "Human in situ cytokine and leukocyte responses to acute smoking". *Journal of Immunotoxicology* 14.1 (2017): 109–115.

6 Nindl, Bradley C., et al. "Perspectives on resilience for military readiness and preparedness: Report of an international military physiology roundtable". *Journal of Science and Medicine in Sport* 21.11 (2018): 1116–1124.

7 Lin, Tzu-Wei, and Yu-Min Kuo. "Exercise benefits brain function: The monoamine connection". *Brain Sciences* 3.1 (2013): 39–53.

8 Marquez, C.M.S., et al. "High-intensity interval training evokes larger serum BDNF levels compared with intense continuous exercise". *Journal of Applied Physiology* 119.12 (2015): 1363–1373.

9 Mee-Inta, Onanong, Zi-Wei Zhao, and Yu-Min Kuo. "Physical exercise inhibits inflammation and microglial activation". *Cells* 8.7 (2019): 691.

10 Calegari, Leonardo, et al. "Exercise training improves the IL-10/TNF-α cytokine balance in the gastrocnemius of rats with heart failure". *Brazilian Journal of Physical Therapy* 22.2 (2018): 154–160.

11 Kim, Tammy D., Suji Lee, and Sujung Yoon. "Inflammation in post-traumatic stress disorder (PTSD): A review of potential correlates of PTSD with a neurological perspective". *Antioxidants* 9.2 (2020): 107.

12 Lavin, Kaleen M., et al. "Effects of aging and lifelong aerobic exercise on basal and exercise-induced inflammation". *Journal of Applied Physiology* 128.1 (2020): 87–99.

13 Khalafi, Mousa, Abbas Malandish, and Sara K. Rosenkranz. "The impact of exercise training on inflammatory markers in postmenopausal women: A systemic review and meta-analysis". *Experimental Gerontology* (2021): 111398.

14 Deemer, Sarah E., et al. "Pilot study: An acute bout of high intensity interval exercise increases 12.5 h GH secretion". *Physiological Reports* 6.2 (2018): e13563.

15 Franco, Celina, et al. "Growth hormone treatment reduces abdominal visceral fat in postmenopausal women with abdominal obesity: A 12-month placebo-controlled trial". *Journal of Clinical Endocrinology & Metabolism* 90.3 (2005): 1466–1474.

16 Gerosa-Neto, José, et al. "Impact of long-term high-intensity interval and moderate-intensity continuous training on subclinical inflammation in overweight/obese adults". *Journal of Exercise Rehabilitation* 12.6 (2016): 575.

17 Lira, Fabio Santos, et al. "Short-term high-and moderate-intensity training modifies inflammatory and metabolic factors in response to acute exercise". *Frontiers in Physiology* 8 (2017): 856.

18 Wedell-Neergaard, Anne-Sophie, et al. "Exercise-induced changes in visceral adipose tissue mass are regulated by IL-6 signaling: A randomized controlled trial". *Cell Metabolism* 29.4 (2019): 844–855.

19 Knaepen, Kristel, et al. "Neuroplasticity: Exercise-induced response of peripheral brain-derived neurotrophic factor". *Sports Medicine* 40.9 (2010): 765–801.

20 Saucedo Marquez, Cinthia Maria, et al. "High-intensity interval training evokes larger serum BDNF levels compared with intense continuous exercise". *Journal of Applied Physiology* 119.12 (2015): 1363–1373.

21 Tauler, Pedro, et al. "Changes in salivary hormones, immunoglobulin A, and C-reactive protein in response to ultra-endurance exercises". *Applied Physiology, Nutrition, and Metabolism* 39.5 (2014): 560–565.

22 Winter, Bernward, et al. "High impact running improves learning".
    Neurobiology of Learning and Memory 87.4 (2007): 597–609.

23 Griffin, Éadaoin W., et al. "Aerobic exercise improves hippocampal
    function and increases BDNF in the serum of young adult males".
    Physiology & Behavior 104.5 (2011): 934–941.

24 Kao, Shih-Chun, et al. "The acute effects of high-intensity interval
    training and moderate-intensity continuous exercise on declarative
    memory and inhibitory control". *Psychology of Sport and Exercise* 38 (2018):
    90–99.

25 Miller, Michael G., et al. "A comparison of high-intensity interval
    training (HIIT) volumes on cognitive performance". *Journal of Cognitive
    Enhancement* 3.2 (2019): 168–173.

26 Smidowicz, Angelika, and Julita Regula. "Effect of nutritional status and
    dietary patterns on human serum C-reactive protein and interleukin-6
    concentrations". *Advances in Nutrition* 6.6 (2015): 738–747.

27 Park, Hye Soon, Jung Yul Park, and Rina Yu. "Relationship of obesity and
    visceral adiposity with serum concentrations of CRP, TNF-α and IL-6".
    Diabetes Research and Clinical Practice 69.1 (2005): 29–35.

28 Krajcovicova-Kudlackova, M., and P. Blazicek. "C-reactive protein and
    nutrition". *Bratislavské lekárske listy* 106.11 (2005): 345.

29 Ma, Yunsheng, et al. "Association between dietary fiber and markers of
    systemic inflammation in the Women's Health Initiative Observational
    Study". *Nutrition* 24.10 (2008): 941–949.

30 White, B. Douglas, et al. "Low protein diets increase neuropeptide Y gene
    expression in the basomedial hypothalamus of rats". *Journal of Nutrition*
    124.8 (1994): 1152–1160.

31 Morgan III, Charles A., et al. "Plasma neuropeptide-Y concentrations in
    humans exposed to military survival training". *Biological Psychiatry* 47.10
    (2000): 902–909.

32 Sah, R., and T.D. Geracioti. "Neuropeptide Y and posttraumatic stress
    disorder". *Molecular Psychiatry* 18.6 (2013): 646–655.

33 White, B. Douglas, et al. "Low protein diets increase neuropeptide Y gene
    expression in the basomedial hypothalamus of rats". *Journal of Nutrition*
    124.8 (1994): 1152–1160.

34 Zhu, Ping, et al. "Cold exposure promotes obesity and impairs glucose
    homeostasis in mice subjected to a highfat diet". *Molecular Medicine
    Reports* 18.4 (2018): 3923–3931.

35 Panossian, Alexander George, et al. "Adaptogens stimulate neuropeptide Y and Hsp72 expression and release in neuroglia cells". *Frontiers in Neuroscience* 6 (2012): 6.

36 Ahluwalia, Namanjeet, et al. "Dietary patterns, inflammation and the metabolic syndrome". *Diabetes & Metabolism* 39.2 (2013): 99–110.

37 Chrysohoou, Christina, et al. "Adherence to the Mediterranean diet attenuates inflammation and coagulation process in healthy adults: The ATTICA Study". *Journal of the American College of Cardiology* 44.1 (2004): 152–158.

38 Bustamante, Marta F., et al. "Design of an anti-inflammatory diet (ITIS diet) for patients with rheumatoid arthritis". *Contemporary Clinical Trials Communications* 17 (2020): 100524.

39 Matcham, Faith, et al. "The prevalence of depression in rheumatoid arthritis: A systematic review and meta-analysis". *Rheumatology* 52.12 (2013): 2136–2148.

40 Yoshida, Yuji, and Toshio Tanaka. "Interleukin 6 and rheumatoid arthritis". *BioMed Research International* 2014 (2014).

41 Hodes, Georgia E., et al. "Individual differences in the peripheral immune system promote resilience versus susceptibility to social stress". *Proceedings of the National Academy of Sciences* 111.45 (2014): 16136–16141.

42 https://www.marketsandmarkets.com/Market-Reports/ dietary-supplements-market-973.html?gclid=CjwKCAiAn O2MBhApEiwA8qoHYeovzbRAw8IbVQvFWQzc8MAA OAQ_xcMRoN58NnCtYXc8ondzPA4l2RoCaLEQAvD_BwE

43 Devpura, Ganpat, et al. "Randomized placebo-controlled pilot clinical trial on the efficacy of ayurvedic treatment regime on COVID-19 positive patients". *Phytomedicine* 84 (2021): 153494.

44 Priyanka, G., et al. "Adaptogenic and immunomodulatory activity of ashwagandha root extract: An experimental study in an equine model". *Frontiers in Veterinary Science* 7 (2020): 700.

45 Sikandan, Abudubari, Takahisa Shinomiya, and Yukitoshi Nagahara. "Ashwagandha root extract exerts anti-inflammatory effects in HaCaT cells by inhibiting the MAPK/NFκB pathways and by regulating cytokines". *International Journal of Molecular Medicine* 42.1 (2018): 425–434.

46 Bansal, Priya, and Sugato Banerjee. "Effect of Withinia somnifera and Shilajit on alcohol addiction in mice". *Pharmacognosy Magazine* 12.Suppl 2 (2016): S121.

47 Herr, Nadine, Christoph Bode, and Daniel Duerschmied. "The effects of serotonin in immune cells". *Frontiers in Cardiovascular Medicine* 4 (2017): 48.

48 Shaito, Abdullah, et al. "Potential adverse effects of resveratrol: A literature review". *International Journal of Molecular Sciences* 21.6 (2020): 2084.

49 Li, Yao, et al. "Quercetin, inflammation and immunity". *Nutrients* 8.3 (2016): 167.

50 Mohos, Violetta, et al. "Inhibitory effects of quercetin and its main methyl, sulfate, and glucuronic acid conjugates on cytochrome P450 enzymes, and on OATP, BCRP and MRP2 transporters". *Nutrients* 12.8 (2020): 2306.

51 Lin, Jin-Yuarn, and Ching-Yin Tang. "Strawberry, loquat, mulberry, and bitter melon juices exhibit prophylactic effects on LPS-induced inflammation using murine peritoneal macrophages". *Food Chemistry* 107.4 (2008): 1587–1596.

52 Krishnaswamy, Kamala. "Traditional Indian spices and their health significance". *Asia Pacific Journal of Clinical Nutrition* 17.S1 (2008): 265–268.

53 Mueller, Monika, Stefanie Hobiger, and Alois Jungbauer. "Anti-inflammatory activity of extracts from fruits, herbs and spices". *Food Chemistry* 122.4 (2010): 987–996.

Part 3: Lessons in resilience from Olympic champions – a masterclass in behavioural science

1 Arnold, Rachel, and David Fletcher. "A research synthesis and taxonomic classification of the organizational stressors encountered by sport performers". *Journal of Sport and Exercise Psychology* 34.3 (2012): 397–429.

2 Fletcher, David, and Mustafa Sarkar. "A grounded theory of psychological resilience in Olympic champions". *Psychology of Sport and Exercise* 13.5 (2012): 669–678.

Skill #1 : Cognitive reappraisal

1 Dweck, Carol S. *Mindset: Changing the Way You Think to Fulfil Your Potential.* Hachette, 2017.

Skill #2: Metacognition

1 Hatzigeorgiadis, Antonis, et al. "Self-talk and sports performance: A meta-analysis". *Perspectives on Psychological Science* 6.4 (2011): 348–356.

2 Greenberg, Daniel L., and Barbara J. Knowlton. "The role of visual imagery in autobiographical memory". *Memory & Cognition* 42.6 (2014): 922–934.

3 D'Argembeau, Arnaud, and Martial van der Linden. "Individual differences in the phenomenology of mental time travel: The effect of vivid visual imagery and emotion regulation strategies". *Consciousness and Cognition* 15.2 (2006): 342–350.

4 Simonsmeier, Bianca A., et al. "The effects of imagery interventions in sports: A meta-analysis". *International Review of Sport and Exercise Psychology* (2020): 1–22.

5 Berthoud, Hans-Rudolf, and Winfried L. Neuhuber. "Functional and chemical anatomy of the afferent vagal system". *Autonomic Neuroscience* 85.1–3 (2000): 1–17.

6 Li, Peng, and Kevin Yackle. "Sighing". *Current Biology* 27.3 (2017): R88–R89.

7 Van Duinen, Marlies A., et al. "CO_2 challenge induced HPA axis activation in panic". *International Journal of Neuropsychopharmacology* 10.6 (2007): 797–804.

8 Telch, Michael J., et al. "Emotional reactivity to a single inhalation of 35% carbon dioxide and its association with later symptoms of posttraumatic stress disorder and anxiety in soldiers deployed to Iraq". *Archives of General Psychiatry* 69.11 (2012): 1161–1168.

9 Vlemincx, Elke, and Olivier Luminet. "Sighs can become learned behaviors via operant learning". *Biological Psychology* 151 (2020): 107850.

10 https://www.tennis.com/news/articles/tsitsipas-secret-weapon-better-breathing-how -can-it-help-your-game

11 Zaccaro, Andrea, et al. "How breath-control can change your life: A systematic review on psycho-physiological correlates of slow breathing". *Frontiers in Human Neuroscience* 12 (2018): 353.

12 Thayer, Julian F., et al. "A meta-analysis of heart rate variability and neuroimaging studies: Implications for heart rate variability as a marker of stress and health". *Neuroscience & Biobehavioral Reviews* 36.2 (2012): 747–756.

13 Gerritsen, Roderik J.S., and Guido P.H. Band. "Breath of life: The respiratory vagal stimulation model of contemplative activity". *Frontiers in Human Neuroscience* 12 (2018): 397.

Skill #3: Positive personality

1 Johnson, Debra L., et al. "Cerebral blood flow and personality: A positron emission tomography study". *American Journal of Psychiatry* 156.2 (1999): 252–257.
2 Fu, Yu. "On the nature of extraversion: Variation in conditioned contextual activation of dopamine-facilitated affective, cognitive, and motor processes". *Frontiers in Human Neuroscience* 7 (2013): 288.
3 Newman, Ehren L., et al. "Cholinergic modulation of cognitive processing: Insights drawn from computational models". *Frontiers in Behavioral Neuroscience* 6 (2012): 24.
4 Power, Robert A., and Michael Pluess. "Heritability estimates of the Big Five personality traits based on common genetic variants". *Translational Psychiatry* 5.7 (2015): e604.
5 Huynh, Yen Nhi. "Who am I?: The neurobiology of the Big Five". University of Skörde (2019).
6 Metzl, Einat S., and Malissa A. Morrell. "The role of creativity in models of resilience: Theoretical exploration and practical applications". *Journal of Creativity in Mental Health* 3.3 (2008): 303–318.
7 Kaufman, Scott Barry, et al. "Openness to experience and intellect differentially predict creative achievement in the arts and sciences". *Journal of Personality* 84.2 (2016): 248–258.
8 Nijstad, Bernard A., et al. "The dual pathway to creativity model: Creative ideation as a function of flexibility and persistence". *European Review of Social Psychology* 21.1 (2010): 34–77.
9 Baas, Matthijs, Carsten K.W. De Dreu, and Bernard A. Nijstad. "A meta-analysis of 25 years of mood-creativity research: Hedonic tone, activation, or regulatory focus". *Psychological Bulletin* 134.6 (2008): 779.
10 Vos, Theo, et al. "Global burden of 369 diseases and injuries in 204 countries and territories, 1990–2019: A systematic analysis for the Global Burden of Disease Study 2019". *The Lancet* 396.10258 (2020): 1204–1222.
11 Santomauro, Damian F., et al. "Global prevalence and burden of depressive and anxiety disorders in 204 countries and territories in 2020 due to the COVID-19 pandemic". *The Lancet* 398.10312 (2021): 1700–1712.

12 Byron, Kris, and Shalini Khazanchi. "A meta-analytic investigation of the relationship of state and trait anxiety to performance on figural and verbal creative tasks". *Personality and Social Psychology Bulletin* 37.2 (2011): 269–283.

13 Bledow, Ronald, Kathrin Rosing, and Michael Frese. "A dynamic perspective on affect and creativity". *Academy of Management Journal* 56.2 (2013): 432–450.

14 Bittner, Jenny V., Mareen Bruena, and Eric F. Rietzschel. "Cooperation goals, regulatory focus, and their combined effects on creativity". *Thinking Skills and Creativity* 19 (2016): 260–268.

15 Adelstein, Jonathan S., et al. "Personality is reflected in the brain's intrinsic functional architecture". *PLoS One* 6.11 (2011): e27633.

16 Käckenmester, Wiebke, Antonia Bott, and Jan Wacker. "Openness to experience predicts dopamine effects on divergent thinking". *Personality Neuroscience* 2 (2019).

17 Boot, Nathalie, et al. "Creative cognition and dopaminergic modulation of fronto-striatal networks: Integrative review and research agenda". *Neuroscience & Biobehavioral Reviews* 78 (2017): 13–23.

18 Martin, Leslie R., Howard S. Friedman, and Joseph E. Schwartz. "Personality and mortality risk across the life span: The importance of conscientiousness as a biopsychosocial attribute". *Health Psychology* 26.4 (2007): 428.

19 Joo, Baek-Kyoo Brian, and Robert H. Bennett III. "The influence of proactivity on creative behavior, organizational commitment, and job performance: Evidence from a Korean multinational". *Journal of International & Interdisciplinary Business Research* 5.1 (2018): 1–20.

Skill #4: Motivation

1 Reeve, Johnmarshall, and Woogul Lee. "Neuroscience and human motivation". *Oxford Handbook of Human Motivation* (2012): 365–380.

2 Clear, James. *Atomic Habits: Tiny Changes, Remarkable Results: An Easy and Proven Way to Build Good Habits and Break Bad Ones.* Avery, 2018.

3 Mankins, Michael C., and Eric Garton. *Time, Talent, Energy: Overcome Organizational Drag & Unleash Your Team's Productive Power.* Harvard Business Review Press, 2017.

Skill #5: Confidence

1 Moll, Tjerk, Geir Jordet, and Gert-Jan Pepping. "Emotional contagion in soccer penalty shootouts: Celebration of individual success is associated with ultimate team success". *Journal of Sports Sciences* 28.9 (2010): 983–992.
2 Pepping, Gert-Jan, and Erik J. Timmermans. "Oxytocin and the biopsychology of performance in team sports". *Scientific World Journal* 2012 (2012).
3 La Fratta, Irene, et al. "Salivary oxytocin, cognitive anxiety and self-confidence in pre-competition athletes". *Scientific Reports* 11.1 (2021): 1–9.

Skill #6: Focus

1 Groen, Yvonne, et al. "Testing the relation between ADHD and hyperfocus experiences". *Research in Developmental Disabilities* 107 (2020): 103789.

Skill #7: Social support

1 https://worldathletics.org/news/feature/barshim-tamberi-friendship-tokyo-olympics-gold
2 https://spikes.worldathletics.org/post/gianmarco-tamberi-my-friend-mutaz
3 https://www.edelman.com/research/competence-not-enough

ACKNOWLEDGEMENTS

To five exceptional women – Shari Levy, Karen Rothbart, Sarah Taylor, Shaynah Crouse and Tamar Bloch – there are no words to express what you have done for me and my family. I am grateful beyond words and measure. Independently you shape and change lives; together your contribution to the world is simply incalculable.

I would also like to thank my grandmother, Ada, who celebrated her 99th birthday in 2022. You stood by me when no one else did, supported me when I needed it most – this book and my journey is testament to you. And to my mother, who has always been the embodiment of hope and optimism.

To my parents-in-law, Maurice and Jennifer Katz, who have helped me to view the world through a different lens; you are inspirational role models in the dedication, commitment and love you show to your family.

To my exceptional editor, Jane Bowman – thank you for all you have done on the book and in bringing it to life. I am so grateful to have you as part of my team.

Finally, to my joy, passion and meaning – Gaby, Isaac, Josh and Navah. In so many respects, my growth reflects the environment you all create. A home of unbridled passion (which is currently that of superheroes), infectious laughter, excitement, endless play, large smiles, warm hugs, unconditional support, care, connection and love.

ABOUT RICHARD SUTTON

Richard Sutton is the founder of Sutton Health and the CEO of The Performance Code, leading global business health and performance consultancies.

As an expert in his field, Richard works with CEOs, leadership teams and companies around the world in driving effective stress management, resilience promotion and performance realisation.

With more than 20 years' experience in the world of professional sport, Richard has worked with top-ranked tennis players, winning Olympic teams and countless athletes, making him an industry leader in advising on performance, resilience and adaptability.

He has a special interest in the genetics of human performance, potential and resilience. Richard is the co-developer of the DNA Resilience Panel, a genetic test covering 13 of the most influential genes that are key in the area of self-mastery and personal excellence.

Richard is the author of the bestselling book *The Stress Code: From Surviving to Thriving* and developer of The Stress Code app, a highly innovative wellness tool designed to analyse and quantify specific stresses and resilience competencies.

Richard has a passion for science and was a post-graduate lecturer for two decades in the area of human performance, potential, pain management, health and athletic development.

His second book, *Stressproof: The Game Plan*, was published in 2021 and provides nuanced systems and processes for managers, leaders and decision-makers facing stress and health-related challenges in the professional landscape.

Richard currently lives in Cape Town with his family, although his clients and consulting work take him all over the world.